PROSTATE CANCER 2.0

TREATMENT OPTIONS AND QUALITY OF LIFE EXPECTATIONS

by

Dr. Nicholas R. Hild, PhD.

with

Foreword Contributions By
Dr. Gordon Grado, M.D.-Brachytherapist,
Southwest Oncology Centers

INFINITY
PUBLISHING

ISBN 978-0-7414-7629-6

Printed in the United States of America

Published November 2012

INFINITY PUBLISHING

Toll-free (877) BUY BOOK
Local Phone (610) 941-9999
Fax (610) 941-9959
Info@buybooksontheweb.com
www.buybooksontheweb.com

FOREWORD*

***Dr. Gordon Grado, a former head of the Radiology Department at Mayo Clinic in the late 1980's, is an MD, Oncologist/Brachytherapist with his own practice at Southwest Oncology Centers based in Scottsdale, Arizona. He has conducted literally thousands of External Beam and Seed Implants (Brachytherapy) for prostate cancer patients over the past 35+ years and he wrote the Forward for the *<u>Prostate Cancer Primer</u>* that was published in 2004 by iUniverse. That book was surprisingly well received in the medical community but, most rewarding was the response from the many men who read the book and contacted me in the years after to share their journey "after treatment"--- more than a dozen of the men who received treatment after the book was published, connected with me, sharing their "follow-up" issues through their recovery, some of whom are still providing regular e mail updates with how they are doing.**

Dr. Grado was the surgeon/brachytherapist who inserted the radioactive palladium seeds in my prostate in September of 2001 and has become a confidant and mentor for me as I have put the research, interviews, and documentation together to publish this Edition, 2.0. The following has been extracted, and updated in part, from Dr. Grado's <u>Forward</u> to the Prostate Cancer Primer. That text is still available from iUniverse.com or from used book providers on the internet.

(*extracting for this PC 2.0 <u>Forward</u>): More than ***One Million*** men have been diagnosed with prostate cancer in the U.S. in the seven-plus years since *<u>The PC Primer</u>* was published in 2004! And, during this same period, more than ***100,000*** men died from prostate cancer, *<u>twice</u>* the number of U.S. servicemen killed in the entire 12 years of the Vietnam War and 20 times the number killed in Iraq and Afghanistan. Yet, the visibility of this pandemic is overshadowed by publicity and efforts to cure other types of cancers, along with diseases like AIDS and SARS that account for only a small fraction of the number of men dying from prostate cancer each and every year!

Depending upon whose statistics you use, prostate cancer kills more than 30,000 men every year. Historically, statistics have shown that, prostate cancer will be diagnosed in more than 220,000 U.S. men in 2012. What isn't clear to the general public is, the number of men who die of Prostate Cancer is not the same population that is diagnosed in any given year: the newly diagnosed men are likely to be successfully treated and live a long and healthy life so do not be alarmed by the statistics! But you need to know that the 'numbers' are based upon the statistical '*history*' which has been used to accurately predict the coming year's casualties since 2000! So, while the rate of deaths from prostate cancer has seemingly stabilized, the <u>number</u> of men dying each year from PC, is not declining---but the number who die are likely to have been diagnosed many years prior to succumbing to the disease---with advancements in treatment technologies, it is likely we will see the number of deaths decline even more in the future, although living with the after-effects (quality of life) of whatever treatment you choose for your PC, will continue to be the "issue" that needs your attention. Dr. Hild has chosen to focus on "outcomes" you can expect from the various treatments in Edition 2.0 and uses the studies and literature that has been compiled from many authoritative and reputable sources to help you make informed decisions about what is important to you and your spouse *after* treatment.

Occasionally, a well-known man gets media attention and the publicity brings prostate cancer to the forefront of medical news. The world knew when former Mayor Giuliani (NY) was diagnosed and, more recently, when entrepreneur billionaire Warren Buffet so, for a brief moment, PC made headlines in the news but, these events usually make highlights for a day or two, then fade from the public's radar like stars disappearing into the rising sunlight. Unfortunately, what the medical community knows about prostate cancer and what the general population knows, are not the same thing: a pandemic is taking place that was true in 2004 and is still true in 2012---we have not solved the prostate cancer puzzle yet! And despite the millions of dollars from foundations like Michael Milken's targeting research on this disease since early 2000, we've barely scratched the surface with mostly enhancing the effectiveness of treatment tools and technologies. Unfortunately, that hasn't made much impact on our understanding of how PC starts and in which men this serious disease is most likely to find a host. We need much more research on the causes and variables that "start" the cancer cells multiplying in the prostate before we can ever begin to "prevent" the disease---and that research is still in need of research funding!

As alarming as the magnitude of the numbers are, the fact that we are diagnosing prostate cancer in younger and younger men *at an ever-increasing rate,* should be sending a message to the general population: more research needs to be funded and more and better communication between the medical community and the population at risk needs to be accomplished, or the situation will get worse.

In the Prostate Cancer Primer (2004, iUniverse), a different approach was taken to communicate as much of the latest information about prostate cancer that could be presented without impediment of medical jargon, as was humanly possible. To be sure, there are books that have been written which attempt to provide men with real life stories of what treatments are available and what worked and what didn't work for individual cases, but most of those quoted in references in this text (see Wentworth and O'Hara for two of the best) were first-hand accounts that are intended to teach by example. This Edition 2.0 (as with the *Prostate Cancer Primer*), cites several case examples where the type of treatment is highlighted (rather than the anguishing story of a man's journey in fighting cancer), and seeks to provide men who are newly diagnosed with prostate cancer with what options for treatment there are *from which* ***YOU*** *can choose.* More importantly, both the upside and downside of such treatments are reviewed and explained using references in the scientific literature---this is where Dr. Hild has provided men who need to know what they should do with the best and most accurate information to help you decide what is best for **YOU**!

The facts and information provided in Edition 2.0, are presented from an authoritative point of view because, besides being a successful research professor in his own field, Dr. Hild is also a prostate cancer victim. When he first came to see me in 2001, he had seen two nationally reputed urologists and two other brachytherapists, seeking opinions and advice about which treatment would be the best alternative for his particular cancer. In the years since Dr. Hild received E-Beam (two doses) and brachytherapy for his PC, he has interviewed dozens of men who have been treated for their PC, with both radical and radiation (External Beam, Seeds, combinations of both, and cryogenics), and has confirmed with medical studies that the "success" rate of the various treatments are about equal---that is, men who received a radical prostatectomy (retropubic or robotic) have a 'successful' outcome averaging 95% just as the men treated with either E Beam or Brachytherapy (Seeds): success is measured in how many years after treatment, usually (for prostate cancer) the measure is 10 years. There is no "quality of life" discussion attached to that 'success' rate and what Dr. Hild has done with the PC 2.0 is to bring you information on what you can expect after treatment---and he pulls no punches in describing what those quality of life 'events' are, so you can make an informed decision about which treatment might be best for YOUR particular (physical and mental) circumstances to allow for the *best* possible quality of life after treatment, for years to come.

"*...at the time I treated him, Dr. Hild made the observation that information available to the average man faced with prostate cancer seemed at best to be convoluted, if not overwhelmingly confusing. The scientific and medical jargon in most information in the medical and scientific literature on the subject, appears to be intentionally obscure...*" Most men would be totally confused if they tried to use it to make decisions about what they should do about their cancer treatment options.

Thus, this text has a few helpful charts, diagrams, and illustrations of prostate glands, and cancer cells, to provide illustrations more details about robotics and radical prostatectomies than the Prostate Cancer Primer did, because Dr. Hild listened to feedback from the men who contacted him who wanted to know more about the treatment options, how they were performed, and what other practitioners had to say about side-effects and (particularly), about incontinence and sexual dysfunction. So there are more of those detailed explanations in this PC 2.0 taken from the doctors and researchers who are performing those operations daily and not just from lab studies that tend to dehumanize clinical studies.

In my experience, and Dr. Hild confirms this cultural observation: *Guys who have been diagnosed generally don't want to see all the anatomical and medical dialog; they don't want to talk about it, they just want an honest appraisal of their options and to get on with fixing it*!

Noted Urology Department Chair, Dr. Fray Marshall at Emory University probably said it best in a USA-TODAY article (July 23, 2003): *"Men, on average, are not likely to lobby or be vocal about their prostate, erectile dysfunction, urinary incontinence, loss of manhood and all the implications related to that."*

Fray further noted that, Hamilton Jordan, (the former Jimmy Carter aide who chronicled his battle with prostate and two other forms of cancer in a best-selling book, No Such Thing As A Bad Day, agrees. In the book, Jordan noted that: '"*Women do better than we do at this stuff because they talk about their health and they network more; it's hard to get men to do that.*"' (USA Today, Jul 23, 2003)

So, both the Prostate Cancer Primer and for this PC 2.0 are precisely that: a discussion of options and treatments, but PC 2.0 is much more, because its written at the lay-level and specifically avoids the use of medical and technical jargon which obscures the message. So, you won't find Anatomy 101 or even a lot of Physiology and Toxicology discussed here, except as it relates to diet and nutrition in the special chapter devoted to prevention of long-term health impacts of prostate cancer. But you will find a plethora of information about what each of the popular treatment "quality of life-after-treatment" can be expected. And that is where PC 2.0 is strongest: diagnosed men need to know the truth about sexual dysfunction and incontinence as well as what kind of pain and suffering will accompany the treatment, sometimes for years following treatment.

When Dr. Hild was searching for answers to his own prostate cancer treatment questions, he found that most of the literature available to inquiring minds (at least to inquiring 'average' men who were diagnosed patients looking for help), appears in places like AARP Newsletters, the Christian Science Monitor, Redbook, Men's Health magazine, Reader's Digest, and pop-Psychology periodicals where the articles don't address the real concerns of (diagnosed) men and seem to be presented as so much milqtoast. Worse, many of those articles are written by non-scientifically-savvy writers and are misleading or, sometimes just plain inaccurate. Most are exploring the psychological issues associated with prostate cancer: such things as *'success rates'* with no explanation for age of men whose rates are being quoted, no real information about what the difference is in the actual '*procedures*' (i.e. seed implants/brachytherapy, surgery, hormones; etc), or details of what a biopsy of the prostate gland actually *is* (i.e. how many needles are used and migration pathways that are left afterwards are not discussed), and probably most important--what *'after-effects'* (sometimes softly referred to as, 'side-effects') will each treatment cause? And, for how long after treatment, which is really a critical quality of life issue that few doctors are willing to explain *before* treatment.

This last one is the subject doctors like to talk least about with patients, and knowing that men are also very reluctant to discuss such 'sticky' topics, the sexual and urinary after-effects are usually handled with a hand wave and a wink, if at all.

In my many years of experience giving papers at professional conferences to other doctors and researchers in this field, I can confirm that the medical community appears to be less than forthcoming about all these subjects. Dr. Hild once told me, *"its as though doctors receive training in 'how to conduct procedures' and let the patient deal with explanations about their physical and emotional needs by seeking psychologists or other professionals to talk to…*" while some try to avoid such discussions completely by referring patients to various texts or literature.

As a physician and brachytherapist for more than 40 years in treating several thousand men for prostate cancer, I can certainly confirm that the medical community *has* intentionally avoided sounding the alarm! Prostate cancer needs to be prioritized for a cure at the same level as a cure for breast cancer is currently being funded; especially where it is the second leading cause of death in men!

The fact that most popular press publishers won't take a chance on a book that doesn't have the prospect of selling thousands of copies, speaks volumes about our priorities. This is *not* fiction and it is *not* destined to be a best seller but there are at least 29,000 men out there (and maybe as many as 300,000), this year who might reduce their risk of dying if they just read the advice in this book:

Seek out multiple opinions on treatment for *your* specific case!

Doctors who specialize in urology and prostate disease will most likely not endorse this _PC 2.0_, although there were several who wrote to comment on the _Prostate Cancer Primer_ (2004) and a few who were even complimentary. But most urologists would rather not deal with the issues PC sufferers want to know most about: what treatment is right for **me** and what will my life be like afterwards?

But, the urologists and radiologist are the professionals who _should_ endorse this book because its not an indictment of them or of their medical practices, after all. It's a long-overdue book of advice that should be on the waiting room tables in every urologist, oncologist, and radiologist's office, as well as in the offices of urologists everywhere. And, in every hospital and clinic where prostate cancer treatment takes place. It is a book of 'choices' and options that every physician should be making available, even if they themselves are biased about treatment options and skeptical about any that they don't practice.

The alarm is being sounded and ***Prostate Cancer 2.0*** is calling all men to respond. Buy the book, read it, then give it to all your friends to read. Nearly two million men diagnosed since Y2K became an echo, will tell you they wish such information had been available when they were diagnosed. Dr. Hild was one of them; his response to the alarm in both the First and current Edition 2.0, of great and honest advice intended to benefit the next million men who are diagnosed. Let us hope they all get successful treatment and live long and healthy lives.

Gordon Grado, M.D., Oncologist/Brachytherapist,
Southwest Oncology; Scottsdale, AZ
Prostate Cancer Primer (2004)

Words from the Author

There are a couple of reasons for writing this Prostate Cancer 2.0 of The Prostate Primer besides the incredible progress being made in the treatment (and progress in prevention technologies development) of prostate cancer. One reason it is important to give an update to prostate cancer sufferers is, the paucity of information provided by the medical community in general, and urologists in particular, to the "victims" remains unchanged from the days when the disease was hardly understood and treated with radical surgery (if, at all) as: "*...the only sure way to 'cure' prostate cancer...just take out the gland, and you will be fine...*"

Of course, we have learned in the 20+ years since that became the medical community's answer, that there is no more "sure" way to cure prostate cancer by surgically removing the prostate gland---what is today called, a 'radical' prostatectomy. In this Edition 2.0, a review of the effectiveness of the different methods used to treat prostate cancer clearly shows that the percent of diagnosed men who choose brachytherapy (i.e. "radioactive seed implants") continues to be as highly effective, or even more effective, <u>for a 10 year period after treatment</u>, which is the measurement quoted by doctors who treat prostate cancer with a radical prostatectomy. Those percentages are above 95% whereas radical surgery continues to be..."*<u>approaching</u>* 95%..." according to the National Cancer Institute (2006). They dubbed the procedure, "radical" for a reason, because of all the choices for treatment, surgical prostatectomy is the most radical!

A second reason to provide this updated Edition 2.0 is to remind all men who have been diagnosed with prostate cancer that---listen up, now(!)---if you are reading this Edition, you need to have the main message of the entire book repeated over and over again because, evidently, most of the men (and/or their caring partners who actually DID read the First Edition...) didn't get this message. Thus, I am stating it here in bold capital letters and it will be repeated again at the beginning of EACH chapter in the Second Edition:

> **"IF YOU HAVE BEEN DIAGNOSED WITH CANCER (ANY CANCER... *NOT JUST PROSTATE CANCER*, YOU ABSOLUTELY *<u>MUST</u>* SEEK MORE THAN ONE MEDICAL OPINION ABOUT YOUR TREATMENT OPTIONS! AND, YOU ABSOLUTELY *<u>MUST</u>* SEEK OPINIONS FROM DIFFERENT TREATMENT SPECIALISTS: SURGERY, RADIATION, CRYOGENICS, ROBOTICS SURGERY; ETC."**

It cannot be stated more clearly than that. Everything in this book is written with the intent of providing you with the optimum amount of information that you need to make an informed decision about treatment that is best for YOUR circumstances. No one, especially not a single-specialty doctor, can tell you what treatment is YOUR best choice, even though some will try to say..."my way is best and the only way for a successful outcome..." or words to that effect. But, few doctors will actually give you advice for treatment in those exact words; rather, you have to listen very carefully to what they are actually saying: they are actually making YOU decide in a way that seems like THEY have given you THEIR best treatment option. But, listening to their actual words, you will realize that YOU have actually chosen THEIR 'suggested' treatment method and YOU chose it without THEM actually saying it IS the best option for YOU. Do you understand???

Here are a few 'phrases' and verbal exchanges that I found in the first edition research; it will give you a better idea of what I am trying to explain:

> One of the first questions that many men have within the first 2 minutes of getting the news that their biopsy was positive is, "...what would you do, Doc, if you were me? What treatment would you choose (if it were you or your son or your father or your ________ (fill in the blank) were making the decision?" Does this sound familiar?

The doctor most often is a Urologist who's 'specialty' is surgery, so the most often quoted response goes something like this: "Well, every diagnosed individual is a special case with unique Gleason scores and tumor percentages and so on, but the only sure cure is to remove the organ and, after all, that is what we do here...surgery...but, there are other options that you need to consider...etc., etc., and blah, blah, and blah..." which goes unheard in the conversation because the die has been cast..."the only real 'cure,'" the doctor said...

What the doctor didn't answer was the question you asked: "What would HE do?" Understand now? He didn't advise you to get a second opinion and, after all, why should you? This doc specializes in (surgically) "curing" cancer and probably does half a dozen radical surgeries a week. What more could you ask for?

The answer is: a <u>*LOT*</u> more! It's YOUR life that hangs in the balance, not his (or her's)!

Medical malpractice insurance costs keep rising because more doctors are being sued and more courts are finding that patients were not asking questions when they should have, to learn what their options are for treatment BEORE they let the doctor "practice medicine" on them. But, because those cases keep being won where juries and judges used doctor's words to show s/he committed malpractice, doctors are now being even more careful in how they "advise" patients. Many Urologists queried in this research, in fact, refused to even answer the simple question: "what is the success rate for patients you've performed radical prostatectomies on over the past 10 years?" One Urologist responded, "...we (surgeons) don't look back for that information. Someone else would be doing that but not we surgeons..." (i.e. ...What 'we' surgeons are interested in is, doing a good job of yanking out the prostate and collecting the insurance payment...but we really don't give a damn what the patient does after they leave the hospital...or, in particular, 5 or 10 years later...we just don't want to know...).

That response, by the way, came to my very own question to the urologist/surgeon who did my own biopsy in 2001---but, I think it's a typical response that I've heard from other diagnosed men in my research---so, be aware: malpractice concerns drive today's physicians; not a patient's future odds of survival or longevity.

ADVICE AND DISSENT

Lest you think that this Edition 2.0 is biased against one type of prostate cancer treatment or another, that is NOT my intent. Urologists specialize in surgery; Oncologists specialize in radiation therapies for Prostate Cancer treatment. These are generally called brachytherapy where radioactive 'seeds' are implanted in the prostate capsule, and/or External Beam (E-Beam) radiation treatments which is a series of quick-burst radiation beams focused on the prostate gland for several seconds, once a day, 5 days a week for 3 to 6 weeks duration depending upon the individual's tumor involvement. These "treatment procedures" are all explained in the book, but a little heads-up here may make you sensitive to how doctors tend to "communicate" (or NOT) about the thorny issues that need clear answers when cancer has been diagnosed.

You need to be well informed about *pre*-treatment, *during*-treatment issues in the operating room, and *post*-treatment potential---perhaps the *post*-treatment quality-of-life-***after*** treatment effects are *the* MOST important of all?). You need to know what *REAL* side-effects are likely from each treatment you might choose to get, so you can choose the best treatment option based upon (not just) % success potential but, also, likelihood of negative side effects, both temporary short term and long term. For instance, if your Gleason scores indicate there is an aggressive tumor cluster, it may be less important to you that you will have potential incontinence (short and/or long term) than a high probability of removing all tumors while they still reside in the capsule (prostate) and so you make the "informed" decision to go with a certain treatment that maximizes your chances even knowing that its likely you may have to wear a diaper for months or years afterward. To save your life, you choose the best (most aggressive) option that eliminates the spread of cancerous tumors outside the Prostate capsual.

On the other hand, you may decide that the risk of not having a sex life is unimportant when compared with a high success probability for a certain treatment that has a high success rate for curing YOUR cancer, even if its likely the nerves that provide sexual functional ability are no longer saved in that procedure. This is what is meant by seeking out your opinions so you get a full picture of what YOUR unique cancer treatment options are.

The point of all this discussion, therefore, is to remind you right up front that there are several different prostate cancer treatment options that may be successful for your specific cancer. The % success for radical prostatectomy and brachytherapy are about the same, while other treatments lag a little bit but may be a better choice for certain individuals. What that means is, getting second, third, and even more opinions than just taking the diagnosing physician's (usually, that is a Urologist/surgeon) is an absolute requirement if you want to improve YOUR chances of remaining cancer-free for a long, long time.

Even if you have to pay for those extra opinions yourself (because insurance companies tend not to want to pay for more than one), the cost of an appointment at probably less than a hundred bucks a pop out of your pocket will yield big dollar benefits, such as…a choice for lowest risk treatment that maximizes your chances of living a long and healthy life…with NO incontinence, NO erectile dysfunction, and a pretty darned good sex life (if those life-style quality issues are important to you).

I Don't Write This To Sell Books

When I first was diagnosed with Prostate Cancer in early 2001, I started doing a lot of research (i.e. it comes natural to a university professor, after all) and what I learned led me to keep my notes and records so that I could share them (and my own opinions), with you. I sought out a publisher that allowed me to do my own editing and make my own comments and suggestions. I am not a famous author in the Medical sciences or Journals, but I do have a long list of publications in the science and environmental engineering literature annals. But, it isn't likely you will hear about this book on Oprah, although it should be a subject she would want to be concerned about since there's a higher probability that black men will have prostate cancer after the age of 45, than other 'people of color' and/or non-blacks, by a factor of almost twice the Caucasian rate of incidence.

But, this isn't one of those books about 'oppressed' people who are struggling to get the word out and need a boost like only Oprah can give. So, you are unlikely to see me or this book on her show anytime soon and that makes it essential that YOU understand the importance of what the message is here for ALL men: YOU have the power to dictate your destiny, whatever color you are. So, since Oprah won't be doing this, you need to use this second edition as your reason for taking control of your own treatment decisions and tell every man you see that cancer comes with options. Only YOU can take those steps and LIVE!

It's OK, also, to get the word out to every black man that they are at twice the risk of being diagnosed with prostate cancer as non-black men, even though Oprah won't be quoting these statistics---or, perhaps, especially because she won't be doing it; YOU can!

Be aware also that, just as you will be seeing news about celebrities who contract PC, you will also see press releases about Prostate Cancer treatment that will be touted as the latest (potential) cure or, worse, news that some medical studies have shown that men are at greater risk just by allowing the screening test to be conducted: to wit, the following article from The New England Journal of Medicine by F.H. Schroder, M.D. (November 24, 2011 OnLine Edition):

> *" '....On October 11, 2011, the U.S. Preventive Services Task Force (USPSTF) issued a draft report on prostate specific antigen (PSA)---based screening for prostate cancer, giving it a grade D recommendation. Grade D means that "the USPSTF recommends against the service" because it concluded that "there is moderate or high certainty that the service has no net benefit or that the harms outweigh the benefits.' "*

That proclamation hit the news wires like an explosion and the resulting fall out was that millions of men over the age of 50 breathed a sigh of relief...thinking, *"...I'm so relieved that I no longer need to get a PSA as part of my annual physical!"*

Unfortunately, what they didn't read was that the study that the advice was based on really didn't show that they were at much greater risk (of what? Having a non-cancerous enlarged prostate? Or of having cancer? Or of seeking a biopsy because the PSA number was high?). What it really was about was not causing insurance companies to spend the $$$ for an "unnecessary" test for men whom the insurance companies think are likely to die of other causes than PC.

But, just the sensational news that men were somehow going to be at a higher risk from the test itself seemed to skew the fall out and that is where Prostate Cancer 2.0 seeks to provide better and more detailed information so men will know how to seek out accurate and truthful information before choosing a treatment (or not) for PC.

So, if you are reading this book, most likely it is because you or someone you love has been diagnosed, so you need to open your mind to taking charge of your destiny. Only **YOU** can make an educated and informed treatment decision. Listen closely to the actual words of each and every doctor you seek advice from, then choose the right option(s). Five years from now, you need to send me a letter or an e mail and tell me: how many opinions did you seek and what treatment you chose, then---were those efforts successful? I want to hear from you so don't let me down---go now, make an informed decision, and live a long and happy life.

Nicholas R. Hild, PhD., Emeritus Professor,
Arizona State University-
E Mail: www.energyprof@gmail.com

CONTENTS BY CHAPTER

Page #

"IF YOU HAVE BEEN DIAGNOSED WITH CANCER (ANY CANCER... NOT *ONLY* PROSTATE CANCER--- YOU ABSOLUTELY *MUST* SEEK MORE THAN ONE MEDICAL OPINION ABOUT YOUR TREATMENT OPTIONS! AND, YOU ABSOLUTELY *MUST* SEEK OPINIONS FROM DIFFERENT TREATMENT SPECIALISTS: SURGERY, RADIATION, CRYOGENICS, ROBOTICS SURGERY; ETC."

PROLOGUE

If you are reading this, it is most likely that you are either a close relative/friend or wife of someone who has been diagnosed with prostate cancer *OR*, you (yourself) have been diagnosed with prostate cancer. Whatever your situation, the feedback received from the First Edition of this book tells me that what you are interested in most is finding the right treatment for your particular cancer…or, perhaps you just hope to be told that you don't need any treatment at all. So, Prostate Cancer 2.0 begins (in Chapter One) with trying to give you the best answer(s) to those concerns that are uppermost in your mind right now.

Unfortunately, there is no single answer that will satisfy each person's specific (physical) situation, nor can anyone answer all *YOUR* questions; men's prostates are only the same in physical structure and function but, they aren't the same when cancer cells are present. Some have more cells, some have fewer and other's prostate cancer cells may already have migrated outside the gland. Some cancer is more aggressive than others and even the biopsy results do not clearly show just how YOUR specific cells are likely to be aggressive.

Essentially, some cancer may be more aggressive than others and therefore require more aggressive treatment and/or a more rapid intervention rather than a less aggressive type of cancer that may be slower growing and perhaps can be allowed to remain untreated while *'watching and waiting'* to see how or if it grows over future months or even years and just require frequent PSA exams to track it.

Thus, one of the measures doctors use to predict the 'aggressiveness' of cancer cells in the prostate is with the Gleason Scores from the biopsy. This is discussed further in the chapters but generally, if the Gleason Score is 6, cancer cells are thought to be slightly aggressive. If your Gleason score is 7 or more, your cancer is said to be likely to be 'aggressive' and if it is 8 or higher, it is 'very aggressive' meaning it is time to do something about it….IF (and this is a BIG "IF"), you seek out several doctors and get several opinions about what your best treatment options are FOR A MAN WHO IS ***YOUR*** AGE!

If the Gleason score is 6 or less, it might mean a watch and wait recommendation is the best course of action. That idea, according to most doctors, may depend upon how old you are: some doctors say if you are older than 70, *'watching and waiting'* rather than any recommended treatment is a low-risk approach that can be shown statistically to have good outcomes---for men diagnosed who are older than 70. The fact is, if you are older than 70, whatever you die from (eventually) will probably not be related to the cancer in your prostate.

On the other hand, for a younger man, a Gleason Score of 4 or 5 may still be assumed to require *some* kind of treatment, although doctor's seem to be less than unanimous about this particular situation. However, for men ages 40 to 70, if the Gleason Score is an 8 or 9, the almost universal doctor's advice is, that some type of intervention should be undertaken in a reasonably short amount of time following the biopsy---although different doctors will look at the timing differently sometimes also, so the question should always be asked: *'on what do you base your opinion, Doctor? (to choose or not to choose to treat in a short time and the type of treatment best for me)?* Again, for those 70 and beyond, that may still be a matter of consultation with more than one doctor---to get several opinions about ***YOUR SPECIFIC*** cancer.

Unfortunately, the CDC and the medical community in general, don't agree on when it is time to do a PSA screen with your regular physical exam---they don't even have a concensus on what the PSA actually means (i.e. at what number should you get a biopsy and, at what age should a man get the PSA?). Here is a recent piece of advice from the Center For Disease Control that muddies those waters even more (March, 2011):

The following information is supported by the CDC on the basis of a study conducted by the U.S. Preventive Services Task Force (USPSTF) of the Agency for Healthcare Research and Quality:

Should I get screened for prostate cancer?

Not all medical experts agree that screening for prostate cancer is right for all men. Prostate cancer screening has potential risks as well as a potential benefit. The potential benefit of prostate cancer screening is finding cancer early, when treatment may be more effective. Potential risks include false positive test results (the test says you have cancer when you do not), treating prostate cancer that may never affect your health, and side effects from prostate cancer treatment.

CDC and other federal agencies follow the prostate cancer screening guidelines set forth by the U.S. Preventive Services Task Force (USPSTF), established by the Agency for Healthcare Research and Quality. The USPSTF finds that there is not enough scientific evidence to decide if prostate cancer screening is beneficial for men younger than 75 years old, and recommends against screening in men over age 75. The USPSTF suggests that men discuss the benefit and risks of screening for prostate cancer with their doctor.

CDC supports informed decision making, which means men talk with their doctors to learn the nature and risks of prostate cancer, understand the benefit and risks of the screening tests, and decide whether prostate cancer screening is right for them. (U.S. Cancer Statistics Working Group), *United States Cancer Statistics: Incidence and Mortality Web-based Report.* Atlanta

(GA): Department of Health and Human Services, Centers for Disease Control and Prevention and National Cancer Institute. Available at: www.cdc.gov/uscs.

Where can I find more information about prostate cancer?

Centers for Disease Control and Prevention 1-800-CDC-INFO (1-800-232-4636) or www.cdc.gov/cancer/ prostate

National Cancer Institute 1-800-4-CANCER (1-800-422-6237) or www.cancer.gov/ cancertopics/types/ prostate

American Cancer Society 1-800-ACS-2345 (1-800-227-2345) or www.cancer.org

Screening Recommendation from the U.S. Preventive Services Task Force www.ahrq.gov/CLINIC/ uspstf/uspsprca.htm

ONE MAN'S OPINION

Unfortunately, the forgoing statement is, in this author's opinion, a total cop-out; the CDC should be ashamed for telling men that "*...they should talk with their doctors to learn the nature and risks of prostate cancer...*"

It is clear that the CDC is concerned about its own liability when they put this burden of learning your options on men of all ages who are just asking for the benefit of the vast research and resources of the CDC for direction---

So, taking the high road here, I must presume that you are reading this because you are already 'down the road' with having not only gotten your PSA results but also it is likely you've been biopsied and learned you have PC. And, you want some answers----so that is what this book is all about; read on!

EMPHASIS IS ON "YOU"

And, this is the most critical point I want you to understand from reading this book: *Every doctor who treats Prostate Cancer has opinions about what **YOU** (the diagnosed patient) should do and the biopsy results they use to make that opinion is the same. So **YOU** need to consult with more than one doctor (i.e. more than one oncologist* **AND** *more than one Urologist, preferably two or three of **EACH** specialty...) in order to have enough facts about* **your** *own prostate cancer to make an informed decision about the correct treatment for **YOU!***

Doctors don't work for free and insurance companies frequently don't pay for 2nd, 3rd or more office calls to get opinions. But, it is YOUR life we are talking about here, so spend the money to find the best options for your specific cancer; it will be worth it when you are able to look back on your treatment decision and know you took time to get the best professional's opinions.

At the risk of repeating myself ad nauseum, this means you should seek out *more than one* prostate surgeon (not just the urologist/surgeon who performed the biopsy), to obtain more than one surgeon's opinion (i.e. there are multiple types of radical prostatectomies as covered in Chapter 3 and 4 later, so even if you ultimately choose surgery as the best 'treatment' for ***your*** cancer, you need to know *which type* is the best for you).

Additionally, ***YOU*** need to seek out oncologists who do brachytherapy treatment (i.e. radioactive seed implants) and/or External Beam Radiation Treatments (EBeam), or both, because each of these very specialized physicians have differing opinions about the techniques and technologies they use to eradicate cancer cells in the Prostate. And, you need to talk to more than one of these 'specialists' so you will know which of these treatments might be your best choice for ***YOUR*** specific cancer.

And, just in case you think that is enough, you really should find out about alternative treatments that are in their infancy that are beginning to find success, just in case, after all that research and consultation, the conventional treatments are still not right for you---it is after all, ***your*** life we are discussing here---so taking the time to consult with several specialized doctors will only provide ***you*** with the best possible set of data with which to make an informed decision.

Notice the emphasis on **YOU**? It is **YOUR** life and **YOUR** decision. Seek many doctor's opinions, talk to former prostate cancer survivors and ask questions---it is **YOUR** destiny so make **YOUR'S** a long and healthy life!

Nicholas R. Hild, PhD.

"IF YOU HAVE BEEN DIAGNOSED WITH CANCER (ANY CANCER... NOT *ONLY* PROSTATE CANCER, YOU ABSOLUTELY MUST SEEK MORE THAN ONE MEDICAL OPINION ABOUT YOUR TREATMENT OPTIONS! AND, YOU ABSOLUTELY MUST SEEK OPINIONS FROM DIFFERENT TREATMENT SPECIALISTS: SURGERY, RADIATION, CRYOGENICS, ROBOTICS SURGERY; ETC."

CHAPTER ONE

Let's Start With The Basics: *What* is the Prostate Gland?

First things first: Let's learn to pronounce the word correctly. ***'Pros'-tate'....***

the word is *not* pronounced with an 'r' following the first 't'. It is ***NOT*** Pros'trate!' (Although, that may be the position you find yourself in if you don't follow the advice here and seek out several opinions for what your treatment should be for your Prostate Cancer!) That word describes the position of lying down and is not remotely related to the gland we are concerned with here, unless you consider that this is the position you were most often in when you activated that little seminal pump in all those wonderful sexual liasions in years past. But, you should know that, if you read this book, the chances of ending up *prostrate* from the effects of *pros-tate* cancer are very small. But, you should know that incorrectly pronouncing the word in public has the same effect on the listener as running fingernails over a blackboard, so learn to pronounce the word correctly....it's ***'Pros'tate'***....and only men (not women) have one!

MORE DEFINITIONS

While we are on the subject of 'definitions,' there are just a few more we need to learn:

Brachytherapy – the word used to identify the process of implanting (radioactive) seeds in the treatment of cancer tumors. This technique is used to radiate tumors with "seeds" that are supplied to 'brachytherapists' (i.e. doctors who specialize in radiology and oncology) for various cancer types, including breast cancer and prostate cancer.

Prostatectomy – the surgical procedure for removing the prostate gland. Also referred to as '*radical* prostatechtomy' because the procedure eliminates the organ entirely, resulting in various side effects that may include urinary and erection dysfunction.

Thermotherapy – the process of shrinking the prostate gland or hemorrhoids with the application of heat.

Cryogenics – the process of using extreme cold to treat cancer tumors which, statistics show, may cause all the same after effects as radical prostatectomy.

External Beam Radiation – the process of radiating the prostate gland with an externally applied radiation beam. This treatment may be used by itself or followed (or preceded) by brachytherapy. E-Beam 'treatment' may also be used to ensure that, where cancer cells may have migrated outside the gland but are still in the groin area, they will be irradiated and eliminated. When used to treat cancer tumors inside the gland, it is usually done in 5-day-a-week treatments for 5 or six weeks duration. Side effects include radiation burning in the anus and colon areas that my cause bleeding and pain for a long time after treatment.

Robotic Radical Prostatechtomy – the same "process" as surgery to remove the prostate gland defined above but with the use of robotics, sometimes referred to as the Vitti process (from Vattikuti Urology Institute, Detroit, MI) or the de Vinci system (www.goldjournal.net). This relatively new procedure reduces the side effects of prostatechtomies, although it may still result in penile nerve damage and/or sexual dysfunction depending upon the skill and experience of the doctor holding the joy sticks.

In addition to these basic explanations of what the various treatments are, (and unlike the cop-out advice offered earlier), the CDC has provided really clear definitions of medical terms that have found their way into the literature and it is important for people seeking answers to questions about cancer, to have these available so they are provided in the following table, for your reference:

Definitions From The Center For Disease Control and Prevention (CDC) National Program of Cancer Registries (NPCR)

These terms and definitions are provided by the CDC from their NPCR web report

(December 2010)

A

Adult cancer: Cancer diagnosed in a person aged 20 years or older.

Age distribution of a population: Number of people in particular age categories. Example: The 2000 U.S. standard population is based on the proportion of the 2000 population in specific age groups (< 1 year, 1–4 years, 5–9 years, 10–14 years, 15–19 years,…, ≥85 years).

Age range: Age in years, grouped in a category (e.g., <1, 1–4, 5–9,…, ≥ 85+).

Age-adjusted rate: Incidence or mortality rate adjusted to the age distribution of a standard population to allow for comparison among populations with different age distributions; for example, rates are age-adjusted to the 2000 U.S. standard population.

B

Basal cell skin cancer: A malignant skin tumor composed of cells similar to those from the basal cell layer of the epidermis. Because of the estimated large volume, many cancer registries do not register basal cell skin cancer except for selected sites, such as skin of the external genital organs (e.g., vulva, penis, scrotum).

C

Case count: Number of people diagnosed with cancer in a given time period.

CDC: Centers for Disease Control and Prevention.

Census Division: Refer to U.S. Census Division.

Census Region: Refer to U.S. Census Region.

Childhood cancer: Cancer diagnosed in a person younger than 20 years of age. Due to the high incidence rate seen in children younger than 1 year old, the following age categories used for data presentation are: < 1 year old, 1–4 years, 5–9 years, 10–14 years, and 15–19 years. See the International Classification of Childhood Cancer (ICCC) for more information about the classification system. Rates are per 1 million when the ICCC system is used. Rates are per 100,000 when the SEER site group listing is used.

Confidence interval (CI): Range of values for a rate that will include the true value of the rate a given percentage of the time. Example: 95% CI includes the true value of the rate 95% of the time.

Crude rate:	Absolute number of cases or deaths in a given population during a given time frame divided by the population in the given geographic area. There are no adjustments made when a crude rate is presented.

D

Death rate:	Number of deaths in a given population during a given time frame in a given geographic area per 100,000 people.
Deaths:	Number of people who died of cancer in a given time period.

E

Ethnicity:	Social grouping based on common national origin or common language. The Office of Management and Budget defines Hispanics (or Latinos) as people of Cuban, Mexican, Puerto Rican, South or Central American, or other Spanish culture or origin regardless of race. The Office of Management and Budget's Directive 15 states that the ethnicity category represents a social-political construct designed for collecting data on the race and ethnicity of broad population groups in this country, and is not anthropologically or scientifically based.

H

Histology:	The study of tissues and cells under a microscope.

I

IBD:	Intrahepatic bile duct.
In situ cancer:	An early cancer that is present only in the layer of cells in which it began.
Incidence rate:	Number of new events in a given population during a given time frame in a given geographic area per 100,000 people.
International Classification of Childhood Cancer (ICCC):	Classification of childhood cancer based on tumor histology. At the time the World Health Organization's (WHO) International Agency for Research on Cancer (IARC) published their first monograph on Childhood Cancer in 1988, Dr. R. Marsden published an annex giving a classification scheme for childhood cancer that consisted of 12 groups based chiefly on histologic type. The classification by Marsden has been modified and is now called the *International Classification of Childhood Cancer.*
International Classification of Disease for Oncology	Classification system used by tumor or cancer registries to code the site and the histology of the cancer, usually from a pathology

(ICD-O):	report.
Invasive cancer:	Cancer that has spread beyond the layer of tissue in which it developed and is growing into surrounding, healthy tissues.

K

Kaposi's sarcoma (KS):	Cancer of the connective tissue such as cartilage, bone, fat, muscle, and blood vessel.

M

Mesothelioma:	Cancer that generally occurs in the chest, abdominal region, and areas surrounding the heart. It is typically associated with exposure to asbestos.
Metropolitan area:	Extended urban area near or surrounding a major city. The SEER metropolitan area registries included in the report are Atlanta, Detroit, Los Angeles, San Francisco–Oakland, San Jose–Monterey, and Seattle–Puget Sound.
Morphology:	The types of cancer that occur.
Mortality:	The condition of being subject to death. When rates are discussed, "death rate" is used to coincide with the National Vital Statistics System data presentations.

N

NAACCR:	North American Association of Central Cancer Registries.
National Partner Organizations:	Cancer-related organizations that value the commitment to successful cancer registration and surveillance.
NCHS:	National Center for Health Statistics, CDC.
NCI:	National Cancer Institute.
NPCR:	National Program of Cancer Registries, CDC.
NPCR Scientific Working Group:	Members are charged to enhance the collection and dissemination of cancer surveillance data. Members include NPCR-funded or NPCR/SEER-funded central cancer registry and CDC-NPCR staff.
NOS:	Not otherwise specified.
NVSS:	National Vital Statistics System.

O

Oncology:	The study of tumors.
ONS:	Other nervous system.

P

Population:	The number of inhabitants of a given geographic area.

Primary site: The location or organ (site) in the body where the cancer first occurred.

R

Race: A group of people who are relatively homogenous with respect to biological inheritance. The Office of Management and Budget's Directive 15 states that the race categories represent a social-political construct designed for collecting data on the race and ethnicity of broad population groups in this country, and are not anthropologically or scientifically based.

Ranking: Ordering from highest to lowest based on magnitude of observed values.

Rate: A basic measure of disease frequency, which takes into account the number of cases or deaths and the size of a population. See Age-Adjusted Rate, Crude Rate, Death Rate, or Incidence Rate.

S

SEER: Surveillance, Epidemiology, and End Results program.

SEER Site Groups: Groups of major cancer sites that are commonly used to report cancer incidence data; for example, colon and rectum, lung and bronchus.

Site: See Primary Site.

Squamous cell skin cancer: A malignant tumor having characteristics of squamous cells. Because of the estimated large volume, many cancer registries do not register squamous cell skin cancer except for selected sites, such as skin of the external genital organs (e.g., vulva, penis, scrotum).

Cancer stage: A measure of disease progression, detailing the degree to which the cancer has advanced. Staging is usually based on the size of the tumor, whether lymph nodes contain cancer, and whether the cancer has spread from the original site to other parts of the body.

U

U.S. Census Division: Geographic groups of states; for example, the New England Division includes Connecticut, Maine, Massachusetts, New Hampshire, Rhode Island, and Vermont.

U.S. Census Region: Geographic groups of states comprising of several U.S. Census Divisions; for example, the New England and Middle Atlantic Divisions are in the Northeast Region.

Definitions Used For Reading Tables and Graphs

A basic measure of disease frequency is a rate, which takes into account the number of cases or deaths and the population size. For example, if a cancer incidence rate is 500 per 100,000, then it means that 500 new cases of cancer were diagnosed for every 100,000 people.

Crude, age-specific, and age-adjusted rates with corresponding 95% confidence intervals are presented in the tables. Age-adjusted rates and corresponding 95% confidence intervals are presented in the graphs. A description of each is provided below.

Crude rate

- A crude rate is the total number of cases or deaths divided by the total population and multiplied by 100,000 (for cancers by primary site) or by 1 million (for ICCC groupings of childhood cancers).
- Crude rates are influenced by the underlying age distribution of the state's population. If two states have the same age-adjusted rates, the state with the relatively older population (as demonstrated by having a higher mean age) will have higher crude incidence rates because incidence or death rates for most cancers increase with increasing age.
- Crude rates are helpful in determining the needs for services for a given population, relative to another population, regardless of size.

Age-specific rate

- An age-specific rate is the number of cases or deaths in a specified age category divided by the population in the specified age category multiplied by 100,000 (for cancer by primary site) or by 1 million (for ICCC grouping of childhood cancers).

Age-adjusted rate

- The occurrence of many cancers increases with age, as does cancer mortality. The age distribution of a population (i.e., the number of people in particular age categories) can change over time and can be different in different geographic areas.
  - The use of age-adjusted rates permits a valid comparison between, for example, one year's rates and another year's or between one geographic area's rates and another area's.
  - Age-adjusting the rates ensures that the differences in incidence or deaths from one year to another or from one geographic area to another are not due to differences in the age distribution to the populations being compared.
- An age-adjusted rate calculated using the method is described elsewhere.

95% confidence interval

- Confidence intervals reflect the range of variation in the estimation of the cancer rates.
- The width of a confidence interval depends on the amount of variability in the data. Sources of variability include the underlying occurrence of cancer as well as uncertainty

about when cancer is detected and diagnosed, when a death from cancer occurs, and when the data about the cancer are sent to the registry or the state health department.

- A 95% confidence interval calculated using the method is described elsewhere.

The following information is from the CDC's web site: December 2010

Note: First among men is Prostate Cancer (152.6 per 100,000); the report and findings are available at www.cdc.gov/uscs

2010 United States Cancer Statistics (USCS)

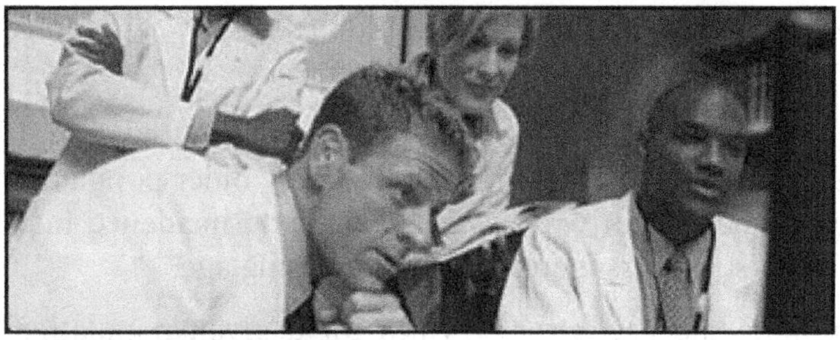

The *United States Cancer Statistics: 2006 Incidence and Mortality* Web-based report contains official federal government cancer statistics for cancer incidence in 96% of the U.S. population and mortality statistics for 100% of the U.S. population.

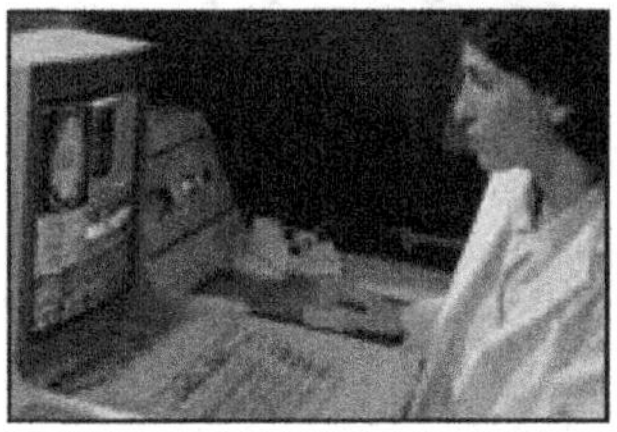

The *United States Cancer Statistics: 2006 Incidence and Mortality* report (USCS) marks the eighth time that CDC's National Program of Cancer Registries (NPCR) and the National Cancer Institute's (NCI) Surveillance, Epidemiology, and End Results (SEER) Program have combined their cancer registry data to produce a new set of official federal statistics on cancer incidence (newly diagnosed cases) for a single year. Statistics from CDC's National Vital Statistics System also are included on cancer deaths for a single year in each state. The report was produced in collaboration with the North American Association of Central Cancer Registries (NAACCR).

The current report provides state-specific and regional data for cancer cases diagnosed and for cancer deaths that occurred in 2006, the most recent year for which incidence data are available. It includes cancer incidence data obtained from registries in 48 states, 6 metropolitan areas, and the District of Columbia, covering 96% of the U.S. population. Mortality data from all states and the District of Columbia also were included and cover 100% of the U.S. population.

Cancer incidence and mortality statistics are reported for 68 selected primary cancer sites and subsites for men of all ages, and 72 selected primary cancer sites and subsites for women of all ages. These data are presented in the following categories:

- By geography: all U.S. combined, U.S. Census regions and divisions, states, and selected metropolitan areas.
- By race and ethnicity: all races combined, whites, blacks, Asians/Pacific Islanders, American Indians/Alaska Natives, and Hispanics/Latinos.

The section on childhood cancer includes incidence data for more than 13,000 cancer cases and 2,000 cancer deaths among children and adolescents aged 19 years or younger. These data are presented by race, sex, age, and primary site as well as by specific cancer types.

Major Findings

Note: The numbers in parentheses are the age-adjusted (U.S. standard) rates per 100,000 people.

Cancer Among Men

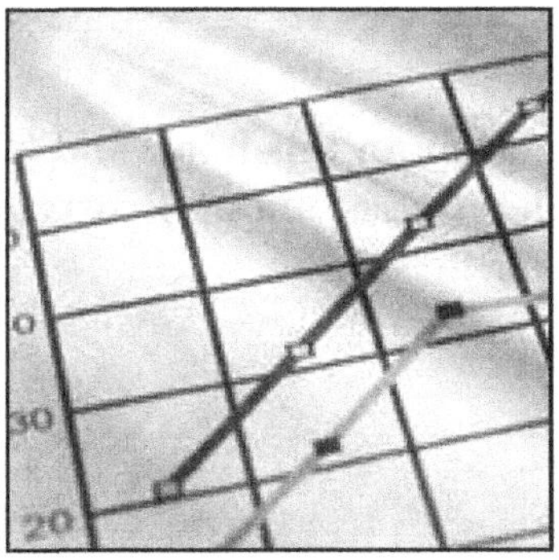

The three most common cancers among men include:

- **Prostate cancer (152.6): First among men of all races and Hispanic origin populations.**
- Lung cancer (82.7): Second among white, black, American Indian/Alaska Native, and Asian/Pacific Islander men; third among Hispanic men.
- Colorectal cancer (54.1): Second among Hispanic men; third among white, black, American Indian/Alaska Native, and Asian/Pacific Islander men.

The leading causes of cancer death among men are:

- Lung cancer (67.5): First among men of all racial and Hispanic origin populations.
- **<u>Prostate cancer (23.6):</u> Second among white, black, American Indian/Alaska Native, and Hispanic men; fourth among Asian/Pacific Islander men.**
- Liver cancer: Second among Asian/Pacific Islander men.
- Colorectal cancer (20.5): Third among men of all races and Hispanic origin populations.

Cancer Among Women

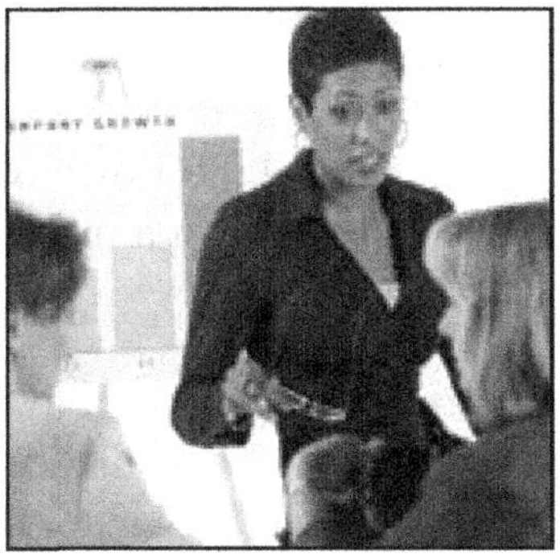

The three most common cancers among women include:

- Breast cancer (119.3): First among women of all races and Hispanic origin populations.
- Lung cancer (55.0): Second among white, black, and American Indian/Alaska Native women, and third among Asian/Pacific Islander and Hispanic women.
- Colorectal cancer (41.1): Second among Asian/Pacific Islander and Hispanic women and third among white, black, and American Indian/Alaska Native women.

The leading causes of cancer death among women are:

- Lung cancer (40.2): First among white, black, Asian/Pacific Islander, and American Indian/Alaska Native women and second among Hispanic women.

- Breast cancer (23.4): First among Hispanic women and second among white, black, Asian/Pacific Islander, and American Indian/Alaska Native women.
- Colorectal cancer (14.5): Third among women of all races and Hispanic origin populations.

Comment: It is interesting that the rate of incidence for men with Prostate Cancer is 152.6 while the rate for the leading women's cancer is breast cancer with 119.3 per 100,000 yet the death rate for both are 23.6 and 23.4 or essentially, equal numbers of men and women dying from those cancers. Yet, there appears to be a lot less information about prostate cancer, its treatment options, morbidity, and mortality statistics than there are available for breast cancer (in women)—

This statistical data is yet another good reason to share the information in this book and to provide as much information as can be gleaned from reputable studies about Prostate Cancer wherever it is being studied; <u>don't keep it a secret, pass it on</u>!!

Know Your Prostate: Ask Questions

Unfortunately, when men are diagnosed with prostate cancer, the functions of the prostate suddenly become less important than learning what the implications of the disease are for the near future. Too often, doctors really don't deal with what the side effects of specific treatment regimes might be when they discuss treatment options. But, depending upon a) your current level of sexual activity, b) your physical health, and, c) how your wife/significant other/partner feels about your sex life in general, there needs to be a frank discussion about treatment side effects that can only be possible if **YOU** initiate those topics as part of the discussion. Thus, together, you need to know everything you can learn about the prostate and how it functions, in order to have a better understanding about which treatment options are right for you.

<u>*The Healthy Cell News*</u> (2002), describes the ***prostate*** as '…a doughnut-shaped gland that lies below a man's bladder and surrounds the urethra; the canal that carries urine and semen through the penis.' And, further, '…it's function is to secrete fluids that lubricate the urethra and increase sperm motility. The prostate is also a muscle. It helps provide the power to expel seminal fluid through the urethra during ejaculation, and works in conjunction with the bladder muscles to control the flow of urine.' In other words, it's the "pump that pulsates the flow" of seminal fluid out of the testicles sac and through the penis so it is vitally important to a man's quality of (sex) life.

This leads to the obvious question: what happens when or if my choice for treatment is to have surgery (i.e. radical prostatectomy)? What happens if my choice is External Beam Radiation and/or Brachytherapy (Radioactive Seed Implants)? Or, what will be those answers for whatever treatment you choose? What are the potential side effects of (each) treatment choice and how likely is erectile dysfunction (ED) and urinary incontinence to occur and over what period of time after treatment? If sex is no longer important, how important is incontinence? Does wearing adult diapers present a quality of life concern?

Answers to these kinds of questions should be a part of your expectations for each doctor that you seek an opinion from as to what your treatment options are. Thus, your understanding of the functions of the prostate and the urinary system it is a part of, are essential, if only for your own peace of mind---and, your partner(s), too.

So, continuing with this explanation…the prostate is only about as big as a peanut until a boy reaches puberty, whereupon it begins to grow to the size of a walnut and stays that size throughout young adulthood. For most men, as they get into their late 40's and early 50's, the prostate begins to grow again in size. It's a normal part of the aging process due to hormonal changes. This is when an enzyme called 5-alpha-reductase, commonly found in the cells of the prostate, scrotal skin, testicles and scalp, increases its activity, converting beneficial testosterone into dihdrotestosterone and causes cells to multiply excessively.

And, for a lot of men, it is about this time when sex drive seems to diminish slightly and some doctors attribute this to the process of beneficial testosterone conversion, although for our purposes here, that doesn't really matter. What we know for sure is, it is this process that leads to prostatic enlargement known as Benign Prostatic Hyperplasia (BPH) or an enlarged prostate that a significant percentage of men over 50 experience in varying stages of intensity.

BPH

It is when a man begins to cope with the increased night-time urination frequency and accompanying bladder pain and/or sleep interruption that the first visit to the doctor usually occurs. Often BPH is diagnosed and, where the condition is thought to be benign, (and for some men who have serious pain and/or start-stop flow issues), a procedure called transurethral prostatic resection (TURP) is performed. In this procedure, the abnormal tissue is cut away from the urethra and, for most men, relief of the symptoms follows. A large percentage of men who have this procedure performed, however, have complications within a few months of the TURP and the procedure often has to be repeated. Doctors think, however, that this doesn't mean that cancer of the prostate is any more (or less) likely. For men who have had a TURP, continued PSA blood tests should still be ordered in routine physical exams and you should know that that procedure really has nothing to do with whether or not cancer is present in the prostate; biopsies are not recommended based upon BPH but rather, are usually a recommendation for PSA results.

But, let us not worry about understanding technical or medical jargon. Let us just say that BPH has the effects, on a majority of men over age 50, of increasing the frequency of urination, interrupting sleep, bladder pain, and other symptoms; even male pattern baldness is associated with BPH! But having BPH is *not*, by itself, an indication that the prostate gland is cancerous. So when your physician does a digital rectal exam (DRE) and mutters something like, '*yep, you have an enlarged prostate…*'

On the other hand---and this is important for you to know---treatment for cancer in the prostate will not necessarily reduce the symptoms of BPH (unless a radical prostatectomy is performed to remove the prostate gland itself), so BPH may actually continue or even increase, if prostate cancer is treated with any other (non-surgical) treatment. In other words, BPH and cancer may or may not be related in specific cases, but a man having both conditions needs to understand how to treat each condition separately.

Or, you may have already had this discussion prior to getting to a point where having a biopsy was what sent you looking for advice on how to treat your prostate cancer (and, why you are reading this book now). But for those who are reading this who have *NOT* been diagnosed, yet are concerned about BPH, and what it means, it is highly likely that your prostate is normal and your BPH symptoms are benign and may or may not need treatment to relieve urinary urgency symptoms---but it is most likely, your symptoms are ***not*** cancer, since BPH symptoms occur in a very large percentage of men as they age through their 50's and '60's. In fact, only one in six men are likely to be diagnosed with full-blown cancer before the ripe old age of 80 (AUA, 2009).

In fact, not all men have BPH or symptoms that lead them to a doctor for a prostate evaluation. This is why in 2009 the American Urological Association (AUA) revised their recommendation for all men over the age of 40 to have annual physical exams that include a DRE and PSA blood test. Cancer can be present, as we discuss in the chapters, and not cause any symptoms for years, so it is vital that the DRE and PSA exams begin in early middle age.

Here is an interesting discussion in a Q and A format, taken from the (NEJM) New England Journal of Medicine (ONLINE, 2011), explaining the use of PSA and side effects (quality of life after treatment) followed by a short discussion about brachytherapy:

Clinical Pearls

Q: How is PSA density used in the diagnosis of prostate cancer?

A. The PSA density (the serum PSA level divided by the volume of the prostate) can help to determine whether the elevated PSA level can be explained by the presence of increased normal prostatic tissue or is attributable to the cancer.

Q: What are the most typical adverse effects associated with the treatment of prostate cancer?

A. With surgery, incontinence and impotence are the main side effects. With radiation, impotence occurs with about the same frequency as with surgery, whereas incontinence is very uncommon. With radiation, bleeding from the rectum or bladder or both may occur and may persist for years.

Morning Report Questions from NEJM

Q. What factors have led to brachytherapy coming back into favor?

A. PSA testing allows for the detection of cancers at an earlier stage, as in this patient, when cure is feasible with local treatment. Second, improvements in ultrasound technology and the transrectal probe allow better visualization of the prostate and permit transperineal source insertion under accurate image-guidance

Q. Which patients are most suitable for brachytherapy?

A. A patient with a small cancer in a small prostate gland and no baseline urinary dysfunction will do very well with seed-implant brachytherapy.

Shhhhh: Don't Talk About Your Prostate!

Thus, the prostate gland is a vital organ and must be kept healthy through a judicious monitoring process as a man ages. Because so little is published about the problems of prostate health, one of the missions of this book was to raise the visibility of prostate cancer and make prostate health a high priority for men of all ages. Prostate cancer is more pervasive in men than breast cancer is in women (See Table I), and yet, men seem to know so much less about it than women know about breast cancer---even men are better informed and more knowledgeable about breast cancer than they are about prostate cancer!

But, its not a topic that men like to discuss; they just don't want to talk about anything they might be concerned about if it is located somewhere below their belt line---and therein lies one source of mis-information: men tend to want to believe that sexual stuff is hush-hush and somehow discussing those parts of the body makes a threat to their machisimo---it just isn't cool to admit they don't know about 'stuff like that' so they don't seek out information when finding out about such things is critical to their future---

And, there is one thing that all men should be aware of: statistics have shown that almost 100% of men will have prostate cancer, *if they live long enough*. So, be open-minded, get regular physical exams, and treat your prostate with the same respect and importance you do to keep your teeth healthy by having a yearly check-up.

Answers You Are Looking For Right Now

Earlier, it was noted that you are likely more interested in what *you* should do, now that you've been diagnosed with prostate cancer. You are trying to get your mind wrapped around the whole idea that you REALLY have cancer and you just want to be told what you should do to keep on living!

Or as one of my friends who was diagnosed with prostate cancer at the age of 44 told me,

> ***"I just wanted to have a doctor tell me what treatment I should have that would leave me 'vertical.'"***

Of course, the answer that *you* want to hear isn't possible to provide because you and your prostate cancer is a specific case that involves your specific cancer cells and your specific physiology that no one---not even the most seasoned and experienced doctors---can diagnose with total certainty that the recommended treatment will give you a 100% guarantee that you will be vertical long enough to see your great-grandchildren.

What you get, instead, is the statistically highest probability treatment recommendation that comes from 10 to 20 years of seeing the results of treatment in thousands of men who've lived

10 years or more after the treatment was done. That is the measuring criteria; living ten years after treatment---studies of men treated with one of several treatment methods who were tracked for 10 years following their treatment, to see how many survived. So, when you hear that a treatment called Radical Prostatectemy (i.e. the surgical removal of the prostate gland) has a 95% success rate, what it means is 95% of men who had their prostate removed surgically, lived for 10 years following surgery.

Coincidentally, that is the same percent success for men who have been treated with seed implants (i.e. brachytherapy) so comparison of these two treatment methods has been shown to have approximately the same success rate, since about the early 1990's. You need to know this, in case you are trying to decide which treatment might be the right one for you. The thing you also need to know is, what were the PSA and Gleason Scores for those men in the studies and that information is not always available to the public.

COMMENTARY

The American Cancer Society estimates that there were more than 30,000 men who died of prostate cancer in 2008 (*www.cancer.org*), second only to deaths from lung and bronchus cancer. At this time, there is a statistical record in every state and several countries of prostate deaths, so if that is your interest, the internet is the best source (although always use the sites like Center For Disease Control and American Cancer Society to be sure your data is accurate).

In a 1996 study reported in the Journal of Clinical Cancer, Parker, et al., showed that prostate cancer accounted for 41% of all cancers in males with a death rate of 14% for <u>all</u> cancers in <u>*both*</u> men and women. In the same report, breast cancer in women accounted for 31% of all cancers in women, 10% less than the men's incident rate for prostate cancer, yet society is made much more aware of breast cancer (and more publicity is published about its effects) than about men's prostate cancer. Why is that?

It's been said that *'statistics lie and liars use statistics'* so it is important not to get unnecessarily sidetracked by the numbers. We see reports and research results every day in the media which contradict and confound medical information. What is important to realize, however, is that not enough attention is being paid to prostate cancer, even where statistics continually show that something is going on. Most people believe the most prevalent forms of cancer for men and women are lung and breast cancer, respectively. According to 2002 CDC survey results, however, prostate cancer is by far, the most prevalent cancer in men, and by a *big* margin. (See Table II for All Cancer Incidence State by State).

Thus, it is clear that for men, prostate cancer is even more of a risk than the medical community would have us believe. And, the percent of <u>*total prostate*</u> cancers is increasing at a steeper rate than all other cancers. Some medical statistics show that this rate increase may track the statistics that show men are living longer. However, what is not appreciated, even in the medical community, is that the average age of men diagnosed with prostate cancer is declining as younger and younger men are discovering cancer in their prostate glands.

As shown on Table I, the most common cancers measured by incidences per 100,000 men in Arizona show prostate cancer is 114.4 while the next leading (lung cancer) incidence rate is 75.8 per 100,000. That's a huge difference! The CDC report shows similar data for all the other states, so it is no statistical anomaly.

Nationally, it is fairly well known that, if a man lives long enough, it is almost certain he will have prostate cancer. At age 85 and above, there is a 90% probability that prostate cancer will be present although, whether or not there are symptoms is dependent upon the general state of a man's health at that age. But, since there is a trend toward more *diagnosed* prostate cancer in younger and younger men, this leads to the question, "what's going on?" From the CDC study that shows the Arizona numbers, it is fairly obvious that there is more to this prostate phenomena than is being publicized.

CDC data exist for most of the other states and, relatively speaking, the numbers are the same throughout the U.S. Dr. David Albers, Professor of Medicine, Pharmacology and Public Health at the University of Arizona noted in comments about the CDC study that, *"one of the things that people don't understand is that cancer is the Number One killer, two times greater than heart disease, for people under the age of 65,"* confirming what we are saying about younger and younger men needing to have PSA screens at their annual physical exams. The sad fact is, however, most men wait until their late 50's or even early 60's before they take serious the advice that, regular physical exams need to be a part of every man's life. And, now, for men, it needs to start at age 40!

TABLE I

MOST COMMON CANCERS IN MEN (in Arizona)*

*(rates per 100,000 people)

Prostate	114.4
Lungs and bronchus	75.8
Colon and rectum	54.7
Bladder	39.3
Melanomas of the skin	20.1
Non-Hodgkin's lymphoma	19.2
Kidney and renal pelvis	15.0
Mouth and pharynx	12.1
Leukemias	11.3
Pancreas	9.8
Stomach	8.5
Brain and Other Nervous System	7.6
Esophagus	6.9
Liver & Intrahepatic Bile Duct	5.9
Larynx	5.7

* Because the author is an Arizona citizen, local media were used throughout the references. Table 1 provides an Arizona Republic Newspaper summary of CDC (2002) report, January 12, 2003

Prostate Cancer

D.S. Kaufman and Others; Massachusetts General Hospital;
New England Journal of Medicine (ONLINE), February 17, 2011

> ***"It is generally considered that surgery in all its forms (open prostatectomy, laparoscopic prostatectomy, robot-assisted radical prostatectomy) and radiation in all its forms (conformal external-beam radiation therapy, using either intensity-modulated radiation treatment or protons, and brachytherapy) are similarly effective for cancer control."***

NATIONAL STATISTICS

The American Cancer Society (ACS) publishes mortality and morbidity data for all types of cancers and produces the statistics every year for prostate mortality, state by state. For 2003, Table II summarizes the ACS Prostate **"Cancer Facts and Figures for 2003:"**

TABLE II

Prostate Cancer Statistics

STATE	Estimated New Prostate Cancer Cases Year 2003	Estimated Prostate Cancer MortalityYear 2003	Prostate Cancer Incidence Rates (1995-1999)**	Prostate Cancer Mortality Rates (1995-1999)**
UNITED STATES	220,900	28,900	168.9	33.9
Alabama	4,700	600	93.1	**41.9**[5]
Alaska	200	†	152.2	22.6
Arizona	4,300	600	—	29.9
Arkansas	2,600	300	130.5	37.4
California	**20,500**[1]	**2,700**[1]	154.3	29.3
Colorado	2,600	300	156.9	30.8
Connecticut	2,800	400	165.6	31.0
Delaware	600	100	**172.5**[10]	**38.8**[9]
District of Columbia	600	100	**256.6**[1]	**53.7**[1]
Florida	**15,800**[2]	**2,100**[2]	—	30.1
Georgia	5,700	700	130.1	**41.6**[6]
Hawaii	900	100	124.1	22.7
Idaho	1,100	100	152.0	35.0
Illinois	**10,100**[6]	**1,300**[6]	154.2	34.9
Indiana	5,000	700	120.3	35.9
Iowa	2,700	400	152.1	33.1
Kansas	2,100	300	—	31.6
Kentucky	3,300	400	141.5	35.2
Louisiana	3,600	500	170.4	**42.1**[4]
Maine	900	100	147.2	33.4
Maryland	3,900	500	**188.2**[3]	**38.2**[10]
Massachusetts	5,500	700	**174.6**[7]	33.0
Michigan	**7,800**[8]	**1,100**[8]	**183.3**[4]	34.7
Minnesota	4,000	500	**174.0**[8]	35.3
Mississippi	2,900	400	—	**46.0**[2]

Missouri	4,500	600	141.2	32.2
Montana	800	100	164.3	36.0
Nebraska	1,400	200	161.5	29.2
Nevada	1,600	200	99.2	32.8
New Hampshire	900	100	150.2	32.9
New Jersey	**6,600**$_{10}$	**900**$_{9t}$	**188.8**$_{2}$	34.2
New Mexico	1,400	200	147.0	33.4
New York	**14,000**$_{3}$	**1,800**$_{3}$	150.1	32.2
North Carolina	**6,800**$_{9}$	**900**$_{9t}$	146.5	**39.9**$_{7}$
North Dakota	500	100	**179.5**$_{5}$	35.5
Ohio	**9,400**$_{7}$	**1,200**$_{7}$	139.1	34.6
Oklahoma	2,600	300	—	31.2
Oregon	3,200	400	154.8	35.1
Pennsylvania	**12,000**$_{5}$	**1,600**$_{5}$	167.0	34.6
Rhode Island	900	100	172.2	33.9
South Carolina	3,800	500	**177.5**$_{6}$	**43.2**$_{3}$
South Dakota	700	100	—	34.9
Tennessee	4,700	600	106.6	37.1
Texas	**13,200**$_{4}$	**1,700**$_{4}$	148.9	34.3
Utah	1,400	200	**172.8**$_{9}$	37.0
Vermont	300	†	—	36.0
Virginia	5,500	700	145.4	**39.1**$_{8}$
Washington	3,900	500	165.2	30.4
West Virginia	1,700	200	138.0	31.9
Wisconsin	4,500	600	160.3	35.5
Wyoming	400	100	168.0	37.3

Source: American Cancer Society publication "Cancer Facts & Figures 2003."
*Excludes basal and squamous cell skin cancers and in situ carcinomas except urinary bladder.
†Estimate is 50 or fewer deaths. State death estimates between 51 and 99 were rounded to 100.
**Per 100,000, age adjusted to the 2000 U.S. standard population.
Notes: State estimates may not add to U.S. total due to rounding.
Bold1 numbers indicate state ranks in national top 10 in given statistic.
t - indicates tie in top 10 statistic.

THE TREND IS YOUNGER ONSET

Dr Stan Swierzewski, CEO of healthcommunities.com writing for Today's Arizona Woman in the June 2002 issue, noted that, *"the younger a man is when he contracts the disease, it seems to be much more aggressive, and if left untreated, will lead to a man's certain demise."* The medical community, at least those physicians who have bothered to think about it, are somewhat baffled by this phenomena and are, therefore, reluctant to publicize information that might be alarming and for which they have few answers. However, it is time that the general public is made aware of the facts because, *prostate cancer rates are increasing at an alarming rate and it is most definitely affecting younger and younger men.*

As discussed before, and to confirm that a trend exists, in 2010, just as in 2002, according to statistics published by the American Cancer Society in Surveillance Research (2001) and Center for Disease Control (CDC) studies (2010), more than 300,000 men will be diagnosed with prostate cancer. The fact that an increasing percentage of those diagnosed will be men *under* the age of 60 is causing urologists and radiation oncologists great concern. Add to this alarming statistic the fact that there has been no known *'cause'* that has been isolated (i.e. we don't really know how cancer is triggered in the prostate gland) and we have the makings of an epidemic in progress.

Of course, if you are reading this, you probably are interested because you or someone you know, has been diagnosed with prostate cancer so these kinds of statistics are less important to you than they might be for people whom you will pass along some of the advice contained in these pages. So, with that in mind, the CDC has compiled some data that will be of interest to men you may know, whether or not they've been diagnosed---and it turns out that men of all races are still at risk for prostate cancer. The longer a man lives, the more likely he will have PC but, just as true, the older a man is when diagnosed, the less likely he will be to die from PC.

Read the following compilation of statistics with that in mind---and remember: you are not likely to die of PC, no matter what age you are when diagnosed IF you make the right choices for your treatment. Or, if you choose NO treatment as your best option---

Ethnicity Is Still A Factor

Table III shows the incidence of prostate cancer by ethnic category. It is up-to-date and current information confirming what the 2004 Prostate Cancer Primer concluded: Black men are at greater risk than all other ethnic groups; Black men should be screened at age 40 with the PSA as part of a regular physical---and every year after that!

TABLE III

Incidence Rates	Death Rates	Incidence Counts	Death Counts	Incidence Population	Death Population

Prostate. Invasive Cancer Incidence Rates and 95% Confidence Intervals by Age and Race and Ethnicity, United States (Table 3.23.1.1) *†‡ For 2005 (latest available from SEER) (Incidence per 100,000 in each ethnic category)

95% Confidence Interval

Age	All Races	White	Black	Asian/Pacific Islander §	American Indian/Alaska Native §	Hispanic §‖
<1	~	~	~	~	~	~
1-4	~	~	~	~	~	~
5-9	~	~	~	~	~	~
10-14	~	~	~	~	~	~
15-19	~	~	~	~	~	~
20-24	~	~	~	~	~	~
25-29	~	~	~	~	~	~
30-34	~	~	~	~	~	~
35-39	1.0	0.8	2.3	~	~	~
40-44	9.2	7.5	22.1	~	~	5.1
45-49	38.5	33.5	74.9	9.4	20.0	20.7
50-54	131.4	119.0	230.0	40.4	44.8	81.9
55-59	297.8	274.8	498.9	103.6	99.2	200.4
60-64	512.6	478.9	819.2	203.4	226.9	373.9
65-69	783.8	736.0	1,154.1	398.7	370.4	668.3
70-74	866.0	818.1	1,189.2	461.2	421.6	748.0
75-79	817.6	767.6	1,067.2	551.9	339.3	760.8
80-84	650.9	604.5	831.6	474.9	396.6	613.1
85+	526.3	489.9	753.2	305.5	256.8	450.0

Table III. Prostate. Invasive Cancer Incidence Rates * and 95% Confidence Intervals by Age and Race and Ethnicity, United States

Footnotes

* Rates are per 100,000 persons.

† Data are from selected statewide and metropolitan area cancer registries that meet the data quality criteria for all invasive cancer sites combined. See registry-specific data quality information. Rates cover approximately 96% of the U.S. population.

‡ Invasive cancers only

§ Data for specified racial or ethnic populations other than white and black should be interpreted with caution. See Technical Notes.

‖ Hispanic origin is not mutually exclusive from race categories (white, black, Asian/Pacific Islander, American Indian/Alaska Native).

~ Rates are suppressed if fewer than 16 cases were reported in the specific category (age, race, ethnicity).

Confidence interval (CI): Range of values for a rate that will include the true value of the rate a given percentage of the time. Example: 95% CI includes the true value of the rate 95% of the time.

Suggested Web citation: U.S. Cancer Statistics Working Group. *United States Cancer Statistics: 1999–2005 Incidence and Mortality Web-based Report.* Atlanta: U.S. Department of Health and Human Services, Centers for Disease Control and Prevention and National Cancer Institute; 2009. Available at: www.cdc.gov/uscs.

All material in this report is in the public domain and may be reproduced or copied without permission. However, citation as to source is requested.

Table III Highlights: Note the tremendous PC rate increase in Black men between ages 45 to 49 (from 22.1 to 74.9 and again between ages 50 to 54 (from 74.9 to 230). Those rates are nearly twice the rates for white men during those same ages 45 to 54. This is a 'trend' that has been consistent over the past 15 years when incidence rates by age were first being tracked and it shows why it is very important for 'at risk' men (i.e. Blacks) need to begin the PSA tests as early as age 40 or perhaps even before.

The other statistic of note in Table III is that there is a large increase across all ethnic groups between the ages of 50 to 55 (from 38.5 to 131.4 per 100,000) and again from 55 to 59 (131.4 to 297.8 per 100,000) which is the major reason the AMA is on record as 'strongly suggesting' that PSA become a part of regular physical exams for all men starting at age 50.

On the other hand, realize that these 'statistics' are averages derived from tests of actual patients over the year 2005. They do not reflect the actual number of men who did not have a PSA or clinical data that became a part of this screen. So, the numbers (i.e. the 'average' incidence rate) in each ethnic category could very well be more than is reflected by as much as a factor of two considering the small sample size from which this data was taken. It is for this reason that elsewhere in this text, it has been strongly advocated that PSA testing should be started at the age of 40, for all men regardless of ethnicity category. An early diagnosis has been shown to benefit a man in two ways: one, in having more treatment options and two, in successfully treating the cancer tumors which are more likely to have remained inside the capsule in the early years where they can be eliminated (before they have migrated outside the capsule).

The medical community has known for more than a decade that prostate cancer has been consistently increasing in the U.S. During this same period, treatment options for cancers, in general, and prostate cancer in particular, have slowly grown as technology has been made available and approved by the American Medical Association and the Federal Drug Administration. Yet, the historical treatment techniques used by urologists/surgeons (even for men under the age of 50) is the same as pre-1990: radical prostatectomy (the surgical removal and elimination of the prostate gland) is still the most popular treatment.

It was widely published in 1990 that former junk bond financier Michael Milken donated almost $100 Million to Cedar Sinai hospital in Los Angeles to conduct research on finding out what causes prostate cancer (to start). In 1993, the Milken Foundation formed CaP Cure, the Association for the Cure of Cancer of the Prostate, which has provided more than $100 Million to hundreds of clinical trials and research projects aimed at finding a) what causes prostate cancer to start, and b) how to cure prostate cancer. Now, more almost 20 years later, the medical community appears no closer to answering the first question but one thing that has been shown in answer to question b): *other options for treatment are available that have as good, or statistically better, long term cure rates as radical prostatectomy* (for men age 40 to 80). The Foundation has also fostered government supported research that has increased from less than $60 Million to $600 Million in 2009. Thus, the Foundation has had a tremendous impact in the fight against prostate cancer---but the fact remains, we still don't know what causes it in the first place!

Treatment Efficiency Has Improved

But, there now is renewed hope that detection methods which predict how aggressive the treatment should be for the man who is diagnosed, will help doctors determine what treatment should be selected for *each* individual---because, prostate cancer cells ***ARE*** different in each individual prostate! For instance, researchers at the University of Michigan Medical School announced in 2002, that they had found 55 genes that were more active in metastatic cells than in less-lethal cells with a gene called EZH2 the most active of all. What this could mean, although not yet studied, is isolation of this particular gene in an individual's metastatic cancer cells, would be an indicator of how quickly cancer cells might spread to other organs in the body.

In the Michigan study, what they have determined is that the *intensity* of the genes' expression, or the prevalence of proteins for which the gene serves as a code, increased as tissue samples progressed from benign to localized to metastatic (i.e. it is when prostate cancer cells have migrated outside the prostate capsule and into other parts of the body that it is most dangerous, leading to higher rates of mortality).

Researchers noted that, higher levels of the EZH2 protein were more likely to eventually get the deadlier form of the disease so the gene may be a lethal biomarker which portends aggressiveness. If the EZH2 protein can be monitored in the other PSA (blood) tests used to screen for prostate cancer, it may be a more accurate way of predicting a patient's survival chances, or at the least, a more accurate way of predicting just how quickly cancer cells might progress, than is presently available. That, in turn, leads to more certainty of treatment choice selection which, until now, is like rolling dice.

And, judging what treatment option to choose, particularly for younger men, is a major concern because, for younger men, the importance of selecting a treatment for their prostate cancer that minimizes side effects, while maximizing longevity, can not be understated.

Currently, of all the prostate cancer treatment options available with statistically similar cure rates, the worst side effects accompany radical prostatectomies. For example, follow-up surveys of radical prostatectomy patients since 2005 has revealed that incontinence occurs 99% of the time in the first few months after surgery. And, incontinence lasts longer than two years in 50% of men who have the prostate surgically removed, while sexual impotence (i.e. dysfunction) occurs in 90% of surgery patients and lasts at least that same length of time. And, those statistics do not seem to change much if the radical prostatectomy was performed with robotics or if it is performed with the conventional slash and peel surgical technique that has been used for the past 20+ years. Such side effects, particularly SD, may appear to be less important to 'older' men, but incontinence is a side-effect that almost all respondents say wasn't portrayed by their surgeons as being a big deal---until *after* the radical procedure was done!

Claims that robotic surgical techniques result in a higher "cure" rate when compared to other treatments like External Beam or Brachytherapy, are not supported in the medical journals over the past five years. Of course, 'cure rates' are usually defined as *'...post-treatment life span of 10 years...'* so this may be an artifact which stems from the fact that robotic procedures for prostate surgery have only been widely used since around 2003, and data on patients who had this form of surgery are just beginning to be compiled.

The literature that does compare robotic surgery to other radical surgery techniques generally shows that sexual dysfunction is markedly reduced in the robotics procedure while urinary incontinence seems to be reduced somewhat, although incontinence in the robotics patients is almost always an outcome for the initial period of weeks and many times, several months following surgery. Again, this would appear to be individual-specific: how long after surgery a patient remains incontinent may depend upon the skill of the robotics surgeon and on an individual's urinary tract's ability to work with the insulted tissue that ties the urethra to the remaining prostate tissue that secures it. Not much is written about this nor is it a subject that surgery advocates are anxious to discuss---perhaps, for good reason. But, you should know that with radical prostatectamies, robotic or traditional, urinary incontinence is almost guaranteed, at least for a period of time, and for some, that time may extend for many months or even forever.

Here again is a statistical note: when looking at the data that shows that ED is markedly reduced, it is difficult to see where the studies were corrected for age. That is, men who are say, under the age of 55 when they had a robotic radical prostatectomy verses all men who had surgery may not be analyzed; expectations for younger men might be a confounding variable because younger men's nerves and tissues tend to heal faster and be more resilient to insult such as might occur in reattachment of bladder-prostate interface tissue. Or, comparing robotics patients with under 55 years of age, with robotics patients over 55, might show where such statistics can be used for men in those relative age categories to make decisions about their own treatment options.

If another cut is made at say, age 50 (instead of 55), chances are that '*statistical*' results will be different still---its highly likely that the under-50 man will recover sexual function quicker than the under 55 man so the question is, how does that knowledge influence treatment selection for the *over* 55 man? One thing is certain: the more data gathered and sliced and diced in more ways, probably leads to more "data overload" for the diagnosed man trying to decide what treatment is best for him. Ultimately, **YOU** are, once again, the decision-maker for what effects **YOU** and your future quality of life. Unfortunately, this little illustration using age as one of the variables to understand, may be an example of when too much information just confuses the issue. But you do need to know about the side-effects of each treatment, and that some of the statistics portrayed are not too sensitive to age, while other's are: sexual dysfunction and incontinence are definitely 'age-sensitive' issues.

When it comes to urinary incontinence, with *every* other type of prostate cancer treatment currently commonly available, there is little to no evidence that urinary incontinence *will* occur---even for a little while---after treatment. Sexual Dysfunction or Erectile Dysfunction, however, is frequently an after-effect that seems to be found in men who's prostates were found to have more aggressive cells and those that were found to be more "involved" with cells being a higher percentage of the gland's volume. That is, when the Gleason scores are 8 or greater, the treatment requirement with seeds (brachytherapy) or External Beam Radiation, seems to be more 'intensely' applied, which might explain why SD would occur. There is little besides anecdotal evidence in the literature, to support or refute this observation, but you should know that, there is a slight potential that SD/ED may occur with these treatments, although not nearly to the extent that it occurs in the surgical radical prostatectomy patient.

More than two dozen men were interviewed for the Second Edition (2.0) of this book, and each one had the attitude that, <u>*compared with the consequences of NOT being treated with one or another of the options, a little SD that might happen was far more acceptable than the potential of not living---*</u> And, most men also are aware that, if ED is a really big deal, there are potential ways of dealing with it---but it just wasn't a priority when faced with which treatment choice they made. To a person, they all said they <u>***'chose life'***</u> and the after-effects or side-effects were not even a concern.

Surprisingly, the same decision-making priorities didn't apply when it came to urinary incontinence. Men seem to have a different vision of what incontinence means: wearing diapers, accidental 'leaking' stains on their pants, the smell of urine in close quarters and their general embarrassment at coping with the daily maintenance of managing their bathroom habits, all seem to conjure a vision that avoiding it is a much higher priority than sex in their lives. So, while there are experimental procedures such as penial nerve replacements which offer hope for sexual adequacy and ED, there are few incontinence remedies yet available that seem to offer hope for a cure for incontinence, at least at the same level as the SD potential cures---

Just Don't Explain

The First Edition of this book wasn't the first time it was revealed that the medical community seems focused on *not* telling you about increasing rates of prostate cancer. Larry Clapp (1997) has written extensively about the foibles of having prostate cancer in a still-available text called <u>*Prostate Health in 90 Days*</u>. Dr. Clapp's work confirms what Dr. Gordon Grado (Southwest Oncology) and other physicians have seen in their clinical experience: *radical prostatectomy does not always guarantee that cancer will not return.*

That means, when you hear a doctor tell you that "*...the only sure way to eliminate cancer is to completely remove the prostate gland---no organ, no cancer...!*" is absolutely incorrect! Studies have shown that the actual rate of recidivism (i.e. return of cancer) for patients who had surgery to remove the prostate is about the same as for those treated using brachytherapy and External Beam radiation. Some studies, in fact, show the 'cure' rate to be around 90% to 95% for radical vs 92% to 97% for brachytherapy treatment, 10 years after treatment. So, the sage advice that removing the offending gland will be the only sure cure should be questioned.

And, as this book points out, urologists and general practitioners have not been the first to let the public know why cancer should actually 'return' if the surgical procedure is conducted properly---which is discussed further in a later chapter.

The problem with Dr. Clapp's book, and one of the reasons more public use has not been made of it, is that it is focused on healing cancer with natural treatment methods, not popular with the traditional medical community.

Naturopathic solutions for cancer is just not a topic the AMA and the traditional medical community may endorse but we have chosen to devote Chapter Six to the general subject of 'alternative treatment' and other life style choices which can make a difference, although we don't necessarily advocate the use of naturopathic methods as a *treatment* for prostate cancer---refereed and peer reviewed studies in the literature are scarce on the effectiveness of alternative treatment schemes for prostate cancer---although other types of cancers seem to have an increasingly encouraging body of data showing that such alternative treatments are gaining credibility. For instance, reputable physicians, like Dr. Andrew Weil at the University of Arizona Medical School, now tout alternative naturopathic methods for their effectiveness for some specific cancer treatment regimes.

The AARP has published information in their April 2010 Bulletin recommending that cancer sufferers should keep an open mind about various alternative therapies that have been steadily gaining mainstream medical community support. Currently, they note that the National Center for Complementary and Alternative Medicine, which is part of the National Institute of Health, is conducting research into a variety of therapies that might help cancer patients---although, few are seemingly aimed at helping prostate cancer victims---studies that are typically funded after clinical evidence suggests a treatment shows promise for a specific type of cancer.

Already widely used in Europe, the European mistletoe plant is being tested in conjunction with the chemotherapy drug gemcitabine in patients with pancreatic, lung, colorectal and breast cancer. No information on this therapy for prostate cancer victims.

Such therapies as electro acupuncture for patients undergoing chemotherapy to treat the after-effects of nausea and vomiting as well as yoga for the same after effects in breast cancer patients seem to offer at least partial relief; however, meditation-type therapies have also found an audience for any cancer patient who wants to feel better about their situation and seeks a group-therapy as a mechanism for having a support group while fighting the disease. This includes such group therapies as those by the popular Depac Chopra and other self-help 'spiritual' leaders conduct around the U.S.

One of the most popular alternative therapies being tested in this general area for prostate cancer sufferers is Reiki therapy, a therapy practiced somewhat like Yoga with specific 'channeling' of energy to join the mental with the physical "internal" body energies to focus healing energy on the particular organ where cancer is centered within the body. A lot more information on Reiki therapy is available on the NIH website and also by searching the web for 'reiki' or reiki/energy. Keep in mind, much of what is on the web is unsupported by peer reviewed studies but you may be sure that the NIH work is one source that intends to validate results properly.

Finally, there is an entire chapter devoted to vegetable and/or herbal dietary 'therapies' that may provide relief for cancer sufferers and, in some cases, have been shown to completely treat and destroy the cancer. Unfortunately, there are no objective or referred studies that are specific to prostate cancer but with all the positive results that NIH is seeing in their studies, we should always be looking out for new data and information that gives hope that such therapies will at least be a part of the solution for eradicating cancer in the coming years.

Interestingly, Dr. Clapp's thesis underscores the main limitation to communicating what options exist: the medical community itself. Most General Physicians, (GP's) are the first medical doctor seeing a prostate problem. This usually occurs because the patient is having urinary symptoms that involve frequent nighttime trips to the bathroom that result in varying degrees of urination difficulty. This is followed by a trip to the GP who administers a digital rectal exam (DRE) which reveals hardening and/or enlargement of the prostate gland. A simple blood test is ordered with accompanying Prostate Specific Antigen (PSA) protein readout. If the PSA results are numerically between 0.1 and 2.5, the patient is given medication for infection and asked to return in 30 to 60 days for follow-up. If symptoms persist or, if the PSA result is 2.5 or higher, the patient is sent to a urologist for further evaluation.

Or, not! Sometimes, frequently with men over age 70, urologists and GP's often take a "wait and see" attitude. The patient is told that, in effect, *"since prostate cancer is slow-growing, yearly DRE and PSA exams will be the best way to proceed. If the symptoms progress, or worsen, or if the gland continues to grow larger (and/or the PSA results increase numerically in subsequent blood tests), then something might be done. But, because prostate glands commonly are enlarged in men over age 50 and, since prostate cancer is known to grow so slowly, the chances of having to do anything to treat the cancer, are very small."* As for the urination problem, a variety of medications are available to help alleviate those symptoms and most urologists are good at prescribing them all! Of course, as noted in the introduction, there is always TURP (treatment).

Just as often, however, for men under the age of 70, the urologist's advice is almost the opposite of "wait and see." And, this represents an even more serious concern where the incidence of prostate cancer is increasing at the alarming rate it is. This book, therefore, focuses on helping *men of all ages*, understand what prostate cancer is and what options there are for treatment. Most importantly for any man, prostate cancer diagnosed early is **NOT** a death sentence!

So, again, if you are diagnosed with PC and you are under 70, you have a lot of options (for treatment) and the likelihood of dying from this disease is slim. If you are beyond 70, the likelihood of dying from PC is also very slim, whether or not you seek treatment! That is because, if you are over 70, your life expectancy is about ten to 15 years more, and its likely something else will befall you before your PC does---but that doesn't mean you won't have side effects from whatever treatment you get for your PC---and your age really doesn't have much to do with what those side effects are or the severity of the side effects; that is pretty much up to you: your choice of treatment and your physical health will be the determining factors that your quality of life hinges on, after PC treatment.

But, just because you have PC and all your options for treating (or not) seem confusing at this point in time, take heart: Southwest Airlines' successful co-founder, chairman, and CEO Herb Kelleher (who was diagnosed in the late 1990's with prostate cancer) appeared at a company dinner where he swaggered to the podium with a glass of Wild Turkey in one hand and a cigarette in the other. The colorful business leader has a reputation for being truthful, blunt, and, at once, thought-provoking. When asked about the state of his health and his cancer (and the fact that he was both smoking and drinking alcohol at the time), said,

> ***"I don't smoke (or drink) with my prostate gland. There may be some men that do that but I never have!"***

It is not the intent of this book to endorse living a reckless lifestyle, of course. It is, however, important to know what your options are, once you have been diagnosed with prostate cancer. You need to know what to do to live a long and healthy life---and, more importantly, what your treatment options are, and what the after-effects of those optional treatments are likely to be---so you can make a rational treatment decision. It is also not the intent of this book to tell you to *'live every day as if it were your last'* as some people advise. Because, in the words of an old high school classmate *(Dick Rullman, Class of 1961, Ottumwa, Iowa)*

> ***"I tried living just one day like it was my last and I worried so much about dying I couldn't enjoy it!"***

So, read about your options, make the right *informed* choices, and live a long and healthy life!

An editorial/opinion in USA TODAY (July 23, 2003) carried the headline: *Prostate Cancer: No Perfect Treatment.* It was written by Don Campbell, a USA Today publishing company board member, who recently had a radical prostatectemy and he had this to say:

> ***"Prostate cancer makes the headlines when celebrity politicians such as Bob Dole and Rudy Giuliani are diagnosed. Macho Joe Sixpack, who doesn't know his prostate from his pituitary, however, often gives those headlines short shrift unless his wife or girlfriend insists he be tested."***

Further, in agreement with the premise of this book, Dr Fray Marshall who is chair of the Urology Department at Emory University noted that,

> ***"…men, on the average, are not likely to lobby or be vocal about their prostate, erectile dysfunction, urinary incontinence, loss of manhood and all the implications related to that."***

Campbell notes that Hamilton Jordan, former aide to President Jimmy Carter, recently chronicled his battle with prostate cancer (plus two other types of cancer) in a best-selling book, ***No Such Thing As A Bad Day,*** agrees: Jordan said that,

> ***"...women do better than we (men) do at this stuff because they talk about their health and they network more; it's hard to get men to do that."***

In the 8+ years since the first edition of this book was published, I have had phone calls and e mails from literally dozens of men (or most often, from the women who loved them and wanted me to discuss the subject with them) about what they were going through---and, about their being less than willing to really open up and discuss their 'condition' honestly. In every discussion, I asked the man to let me know about what treatment they chose and to give me some feedback about the after-effects they experienced afterwards and one thing I know is this: *every* man I spoke to "pre-treatment" was uncomfortable with even talking about issues like SD and incontinence, even to the extent that they hesitated to use the words and to describe their 'intimate' details of their sexual and/or urinary habits so we could come to some common areas of agreement on what they felt was important to them.

But, when those same men who called me or e mailed me in the "post-treatment" years discussed their lives after treatment, they were totally different. To a person, each of them were very verbal and outgoing about the 'conditions' they had experienced both sexually and in their bodily functions (or lack thereof). There was obvious candor in their voices but, at the same time, it was apparent that they had become accustomed to discussing all of the little details about the formerly taboo subjects ("pre-treatment") that PC imbues, and in some cases, angry about not seeking enough different doctor's opinions about their options. But, all of them who contacted me "post-treatment" were unanimous in their opinions that prostate cancer specialists are mostly poor communicators, when it comes to offering good, clear analysis and explanations of the things men need to know.

So, in this second edition, I have tried to be sensitive to just how little information is publicly available (i.e. that is, information which is highlighted and unavoidable) about prostate cancer and how important it is for men who have prostate problems **NOT** to ignore the plethora of information that is now available about treatment options for decision-making. And, most importantly, to reemphasize that it is **YOU** who needs to visit and seek consultation from several urologists, oncologists, and treatment experts: only **YOU** can be responsible for choosing the best treatment for YOUR prostate cancer.

THE OSTRICH PRINCIPLE

The popular press is slowly recognizing that men, indeed, are different than women in more than the obvious ways: they don't read as much, and certainly not materials that they aren't already interested in. When they talk over beers at the pub, they avoid medical or sexual topics except as it relates to their prowess, but they especially avoid their own physical conditions. Most men, we realize, practice the Ostrich Principle: putting their head in the sand. They would rather not talk about themselves and hope that cancer is something they never have to face. Thus, most of them figure that, if they don't talk about it, they won't get it and they won't have to deal with it.

So, we need to make general health information available in different ways than we do for women. This is even more true for men in their early 40's who need to include PSA tests in their annual physical exams. Thus, this book speaks to that issue, generally, and to men, specifically about prostate health. Share this with every man you know and we might make a reduction in that 29,000 who will die from prostate cancer next year.

Finally, for additional support for the idea that early screening should begin in men at the age of 35, the very reputable and internationally acclaimed Southwest College of Naturopathic Medicine & Health made a plea in their winter issue 2003 SCNM Newsletter for men to take care of their prostate health starting at an early age. For men in higher risk categories (i.e. family history, black men), they advise starting PSA screenings at age 25, citing the recent New York postmortem study which found undiagnosed PC in men in their early twenties.

So, the medical community seems to be in agreement: PSA testing should begin at an earlier age than has previously been stated publicly. For our purposes here, all the evidence suggests that, at least by age 45, every man should have PSA screening along with a regular physical exam. For high risk men, we suggest starting that at least ten years earlier, by age 35 and certainly no later than age 40, in order for diagnosis and treatment be effected while cancer tumors are still contained inside the prostate gland.

And, remember: Most men have <u>no</u> symptoms, even at ages of 70 or 80, so the PSA screening is, today, the most likely source of information that will mean the difference between making choices that allow for living a long and healthy life.

NEW TESTS; NEW HOPE

And, just in case you are that magical age of 70 or older and you've received the biopsy results that indicate you need to make a decision: what treatment; no treatment? There is a new option that has just been a host of newer imaging technologies that have shown promise for better making a better diagnosis of cancer cells in the prostate. Dr. Duke Bahn at the Prostate Institute of America in Ventura California uses sonogram images in concert with those obtained by the Transrectal Ultrasound Probe (TRUS) whereby pictures are taken of the prostate to identify the size and location of tumors. The pictures are then measured against the PSA readout and the biopsy results, to detect variations in the color-Doppler sonogram. This procedure should give the over-70 man another option for data gathering before deciding on a particular treatment regime.

Another test being developed by Dr. David Crawford at the University of Colorado medical school is a sophisticated genetic testing procedure that provides a 3-D mapping that provides a better image of the affected area while giving a better view of the RNA (messenger cells inside DNA), while helping to reveal a tumor's 'danger' or aggressiveness quotient. Again, advancement in imaging technologies going forward will allow for better analysis and better decision-making for the diagnosed man.

Advancement of technologies that allow better imaging will benefit all diagnosed men, no matter what age they are when the biopsy results are bad news. But, particularly for men over the age of 70, the 'wait and watch option becomes more likely the best choice with more sophisticated tools moving from the research labs to the imaging centers.

What the Medical Community Knows

The first thing the General Practitioner (GP) usually identifies from the DRE (digital rectal exam) in routine physical examinations is BPH (benign prostatic hyperplasia). This is the noncancerous prostate enlargement and/or prostatitis (inflamed prostate) that most men over the age of 50 experience. But, BPH is usually not a big concern unless it causes the patient to have symptoms (discussed later). What most men hear at the physical exam from the GP is, *"your prostate is enlarged and we will watch it over the next 6 to 12 months. If you have 'symptoms' later, we will do another PSA and go from there."* And, *"by the way, don't worry. It's* 'usually' *benign!"* This is where we first hear the term, *'watchful waiting'* used. And where most men really start to worry!

If PSA results are in the high range, say 3.0 to 3.5, the GP may advise the patient to see a urologist for further evaluation. In today's litigious world, no primary care physician likes to take chances with mis-diagnosing a problem that might be as serious as prostate cancer. Because urologists conduct digital rectal exams (DRE) frequently, they tend to have a much better "feel" for prostates (pun intended) and their diagnosis of what problem the patient may have is usually much more accurate than the General Practitioner (GP). Still, the urologist will usually request that more than one PSA (blood test result) be taken before identifying and diagnosing the problem completely.

The PSA or prostate specific antigen is a measure, in nanograms per milliliter, of the blood content of a protein known to be produced by the prostate gland , *sort of* in response to cancer cells being formed or proliferating...*sort of.*

Historically, if PSA results are lower than 4.0 (nanograms per milliliter), most urologists (and GP's) will have a 'wait and see' attitude, although they may want another PSA in cases where the PSA result is between 2.5 and 4.0, just to see if its stable or if it is rising. But, remember that PSA levels only estimate how *likely* a man is to have prostate cancer, although it does not always *'predict'* cancer is present. So, different doctors might approach the diagnostics differently; its why we recommend getting more than one opinion when borderline PSA results are consistent over time, before you get a biopsy.

A study published in the Journal of the American Medicine Association (JAMA), in July, 2003 found that men, particularly men under age 50, who had PSA results of less than 2.9, were still at risk. The results indicated that ***not screening men with PSA's between 2.4 and 2.9 resulted in missing cancer in as many as 60%*** of those who were retested. This is particularly alarming when you consider that biopsies are usually not recommended unless PSA's are greater than (about) 4.0, in most men.

An editorial in the same JAMA issue recommended "wait and watch" for those men, somewhat contradicting the authors of the study, all of which leads to further confusion for the man whose PSA is in that 'gray' range 2.5 to 3.9. Thus, its no wonder that men don't pursue second and third opinions when their diagnosis is positive! But, it is worth noting that this same man had elevated PSA's five years later, and his cancer had metastasized into his kidney. At this writing, he continues to undergo treatment.

Some studies have shown that as many as 25% of men diagnosed with prostate cancer have a low PSA (NCCN, 2001). In one case known personally to the authors of this book, a 44 year old man in Phoenix, Arizona had increasingly severe symptoms of night time urination problems over 6 to 8 months before going for a DRE and PSA evaluation. Two GP's and two urologists said he had *'early'* BPH and evaluated consistently low PSA results (i.e. less than 0.8!) to mean 'wait and watch' with *"not even the slight possibility of cancer being present"* as stated by one doctor. Subsequent evaluation at Cedars Siani Hospital revealed almost total tumor involvement in the young man's prostate and immediate surgery was recommended (Cedars, 2001).

Interestingly, a recent study undertaken at the Oregon Health and Science University Cancer Institute demonstrates the confused state of information and "mixed-messages" that are provided about prostate cancer to the general public. In a study that looked at more than 1,200 men with PSA levels ranging from 4 to 10 who had biopsies between 1993 and 2000, the Director of urologic oncology at the Portland Veterans Affairs Medical Center Dr. Mark Garzotto discussed the findings in the popular press.

After a man has the PSA result that the urologist or GP says is in the high range (i.e.usually, above 2.5) but not statistically different than previous PSA results (taken over several months time), the doctor is likely to conclude that *"just watching it"* (i.e. watchful waiting) for a few months is the best course of action. Medication might be prescribed for the urinary symptoms, or, in the case of a patient that had no urinary symptoms but whose PSA was in the high range in a routine physical exam, the doctor might request another PSA in 30 to 60 days. Or, as in the case where the PSA appears to be climbing slowly over three or four month's PSA tests, the option of doing a biopsy on the prostate might be discussed.

Good urologists will not "prescribe" a biopsy but, rather, *suggest* to the patient that it is his choice: a biopsy, they will be advised, however, will be definitive almost 100% of the time… *"**almost**"*...

But, the choice is clearly left to the patient whether or not to actually have a biopsy done because biopsies (unbeknown to the patient) carry a risk that the urologist does not want to be liable for, of spreading cancer cells that are otherwise "contained" in the prostate. More about this later.

As discussed before, a urologist also may say that, because prostate cancer is *"slow growing,"* there is plenty of time to decide whether a biopsy is warranted. Unfortunately, that conclusion, while being statistically accurate, is based on the history of prostate cancer growth in men over 70 where life expectancy is short (i.e. average lifetime is 76 years) and men usually die from some other cause (Schachter, World Health OnLine, 2002) For younger men who face the possibility of cancer, getting a biopsy sooner, rather than later, may be crucial to treatment while the cancer cells are still contained in the prostate gland (and have not migrated to other parts of the body).

Cancer indicators, PSA, Biopsies and Gleason Scores

The procedure for conducting a biopsy of the prostate gland incorporates the use of hollow needles inserted into the prostate which extract tissue samples, usually 6 to 8 in number, which are sent to a laboratory where they are evaluated for cancer cells. This almost painless procedure is usually conducted in the urologist's office using a computer probe inserted up the rectal canal to map the prostate. The urologist then utilizes the computer image in snaking the needle device up the rectal canal where s/he inserts and removes the needles to extract tissue for laboratory evaluation. "*Extract*" is the operative word: the procedure actually tears or rips the tiny tissue culture from the gland as it is withdrawn. And, because the urethra winds its way right through the prostate gland, there are bleeding issues that manifest themselves in the urine for several hours, and sometimes, days, afterwards. This is, however, normal and should clear up in a day or two, at most.

What is important to know about this procedure, however, is that the needle insertion/retraction pathway is left from inside the prostate to the outside of the gland, whereby any cancer cells present, ***might*** be able to migrate and make their way into other parts of the body. This is the "biopsy risk" that urologists do not like to discuss that was mentioned before. Unfortunately, at this time, there are not good alternatives to this procedure for definitively learning if cancer is present in the prostate gland.

AFTER THE BIOPSY: If the results are positive

Urologists who do the needle biopsies know the probability of cancer cells migrating through this procedure is low but they prefer that patients not know about it at all. When biopsy results confirm that cancer cells are present, a radical prostatectomy (i.e. surgical procedure to remove the prostate gland) is frequently recommended by the urologist and there is usually little discussion about the probability that the cancer might metasticize at a later time. In fact, many doctors tell patients that surgically removing the prostate gland is the *only* sure way to eliminate the cancer. Thus, patients who choose to have a radical prostatectomy and then find some years later that their cancer has metastacized (returned) elsewhere in their body may never know that the biopsy they had years before was possibly the way their cancer spread. This would be the *"horse was already out of the barn"* corollary urologists/surgeons use for why cancer reappeared after the prostate gland was removed!

It is for this reason that patients should not wait too long after a biopsy to decide on what treatment should be done. This is true no matter what treatment option, including non-surgical procedures, is chosen since the migration pathways are open from the needle biopsy procedure the moment the biopsies are extracted from inside the prostate gland. Plus, consider that the needles---every one of them---pierce the outer layers of the gland on their way in, and on their way back out. So if any cancer cells are laying at the surface, the needle extraction can immediately carry those cancer cells outside the capsule where they can begin to spread to lymph nodes in the groin, even before any treatment option is taken.

It can be estimated, although not statistically, a significant percentage of patients who have had radical surgery and learned some years later that their cancer had returned and was now in other parts of the body, was spread by this very biopsy procedure. Urologists will never admit to that possibility (for obvious liability reasons), but post-surgery biopsies that showed highly involved cancer cells at or near the surface layers, are high-risk for metastasis. However, there are few data or references in the literature to show just how many patients who had later metastasis were shown to have this condition in their prostate autopsy at the time of surgery. It is a study no one seems to want to do.

Patients choosing to seek other medical opinions about treatment options generally find out from oncologist and radiologists who specialize in prostate cancer treatment, that the risk of the biopsy pathway needs to be followed quickly by external beam radiation treatment(s) so that the migration is stemmed before or just after it reaches the outside layers of the gland. Even for men who choose surgery, or radical prostatectomy, external beam radiation might be recommended to kill cancer cells outside but in the general area of the prostate gland before surgery or at the same time brachytherapy is performed. The urologist/surgeon is oftentimes reluctant to make such a recommendation, fearing opening up liability issues that might be difficult to defend if cancer later returns after treatment, years later. (See also a later discussion about a 2003 Mayo Clinic study that deals with this topic)

Just as often, men being the reluctant animal they are to discuss anything as personal as medical problems with their *"sexual systems,"* would rather trust the advice of the urologist and not seek second or third opinions about treatment options. That is why, about 60% to 80% of the time, surgery is recommended and no other opinions are sought by the patient. Men just want to get the "*problem*" fixed and get on with their lives with no embarrassing "*personal*" discussions---certainly not with complete strangers (i.e. other doctors). So, just remember: it is YOUR life; it is YOUR decision. Get more opinions!

Those are all reasons why proper communication with the general population about the increasingly large numbers of prostate cancers diagnosed and the misinformation (or intentional lack of it) being given out by the medical community warrants a critical look. It is to this end that this Second Edition (2.0) has compiled the resources and data that are intended to enlighten men who are concerned about their prostate health and why there were follow-up interviews with men who were quoted in the First Edition.

And, it is the diagnosed man who needs to know the most about this very gray area of cancer treatment, even though the foregoing discussion focus' on how a man actually gets diagnosed (i.e. via a biopsy), there are important messages to be learned for everyone: seeking second and third opinions is something that it is never too late to do---unless you've already had one of the treatments for your PC. But, even then, if you are reading this book, there are probably some issues that you may want to learn more about and, as with the diagnosed man seeking treatment options, you can also seek opinions about your current PC outcomes. Most brachytherapists actually treat a lot of post-radical prostatectomy patients when PSAs are found to be on the rise---so, just knowing you do have post-surgical options when things didn't work out as planned, should give you incentive to learn all you can; you do have more treatment options than you might think!

AFTER THE BIOPSY: When Results Are Negative

It is just as important to know what it means to get a "negative" biopsy result. Generally, a low PSA result (i.e. a numerical result less than 3.0) will not be considered a potential problem and the examining physician may recommend that no biopsy be performed. *"Just watch it for six months and do another PSA with DRE..."* is a typical recommendation. However, if the patient is having classic symptoms of frequent night-time trips to the bathroom and the prostate is enlarged and/or feels "hard" to the touch in the DRE, a biopsy may be recommended when PSA would not otherwise indicate that a potential problem exists.

Whenever a biopsy procedure is conducted, the cautionary information provided previously should be heeded; if cancer cells are present (even microscopic-sized cells), there is an increased risk that they may be provided a pathway outside the gland via the needle paths in the biopsy. Where those cells might not have been a problem inside the gland for years (or perhaps, never), once allowed to migrate outside to other parts of the body, microscopic cancer cells represent a greater risk of full-blown carcinogenicity in other parts of the body.

There are cases also where men have had PSA results on subsequent examinations of less than 1.0 but the symptoms (enlarged gland, hard surfaces, frequent bathroom urination trips; etc) were so overwhelming that a biopsy revealed cancer in the prostate was present. Thus, a "normal" PSA does not always mean that results are "negative" and the doctor should consult with men who find themselves in this situation to determine what steps should be taken. It is frequently the case that the urologist recommends a "wait and see" period before repeating the tests (including biopsies that have been negative). A man finding himself in this situation should **DEFINITELY** seek second and third opinions from <u>other</u> urologists and radiologists who specialize in prostate treatment.

NEGATIVE BIOPSY RESULTS: Does It Mean Cancer Is ***<u>NOT</u>*** Present?

There are also many documented cases of men having all the symptoms who have a biopsy performed, only to reveal that no cancer cells were detected. Even when PSA results are sometimes ten, twenty or higher, when the biopsy results did not find cancer cells present, what normally is advised by the physicians is, wait and watch then have a PSA again in six months or a year. Unfortunately, in case after case, when the patient returns with the same (or statistically similar numerical) PSA result in six months, another biopsy is recommended...again!

There are men who have had this occur over a three to five year period and had a biopsy each subsequent time, only to receive negative results. But, the prostate gland, after having more than a dozen or two needle biopsies, is scarred and even a higher risk of transporting microscopic cancer cells outside the gland with *<u>no</u> diagnostic method of learning if that is happening or not.* In most of the cases reviewed for this book where this situation has occurred, ultimate MRI and PET scans showed the presence of tumor(s) in the prostate gland, and, sometimes in the groin-lymph glands, even where the biopsy results were still considered to be negative.

SUMMARY

Most men are reluctant to go to doctors with problems that they are having in those "unmentionable" places on their bodies. When it comes to the prostate gland, men are even less inclined to seek medical help, fearing the embarrassment of their perceived "situation" will be humiliating. Thus, problems with frequent and incomplete night time urination, discomfort in the penis or rectal areas, or sexual dysfunction are likely to be ignored until there seems to be no other way to get relief. By then, men who find out they have an enlarged prostate gland and an abnormally high PSA, just want to get a "fix" for the problem, and live a normal life again. The options for prostate cancer sufferers, however, are more than just radical prostatectomy and getting second and third medical opinions is a key to making the right therapy choice.

CHAPTER TWO

In this chapter, you will learn about........

Diagnosis and Prognosis:
What the studies are showing: Updated to 2010

Most Common Treatment Options Today

What surgery and prostate gland removal mean

What External Beam Radiation can and can not do

What Brachytherapy (Radioactive Seed Implants) can and can not do

Cancer indicators, PSA, Biopsies and Gleason Scores

Other Therapies
Hormonal Therapy

"IF YOU HAVE BEEN DIAGNOSED WITH CANCER (ANY CANCER... NOT *ONLY* PROSTATE CANCER, YOU ABSOLUTELY *MUST* SEEK MORE THAN ONE MEDICAL OPINION ABOUT YOUR TREATMENT OPTIONS! AND, YOU ABSOLUTELY *MUST* SEEK OPINIONS FROM DIFFERENT TREATMENT SPECIALISTS: SURGERY, RADIATION, CRYOGENICS, ROBOTICS SURGERY; ETC."

INTRODUCTION

Numerous urologists who do needle placements (only) for radiologists who insert radiation seeds in the treatment known as brachytherapy, will tell you that they don't keep statistics on patients. They will tell you, *"that it's the Radiologist/Oncologist who wants to know..."* the success rate. When you inquire at hospitals where radical prostatectomies are performed, you will find that the statistics are not available (except to need-to-know doctors). And, this is just an extension of the problem discussed before: communicating to the patient community is pretty much restricted to whatever doctors want (or the AMA policy at the moment).

For this book, therefore, we used studies and literature that were taken from public domain sites on the internet, clinics that do prostate cancer research and treatment, and the very large (and well documented) data base of Southwest Oncology which consists of more than 7000 prostate cancer patients. In addition, after the release of the First Edition, interviews were conducted with men who were treated to determine their current state of (prostate) health. Thus, what you read about here is real-world, timely, up-to-date (for the period 2003-2011), and is intentionally written at the lay-public level with as few medical jargon terms as possible.

It is anticipated, also, as it proved to be with the First Edition, that our biggest critics will be from the medical community. But, we encourage debate and, most of all, for men of all ages, the medical community needs to be more forthcoming on this increasingly controversial problem. If this Edition 2.0 succeeds in providing options to even a handful of men, we have fulfilled our goal---and the First Edition did just that!

DIAGNOSIS AND PROGNOSIS: What the studies are showing

When we looked back at the thousands of brachytherapy patients treated by Dr. Grado and Dr. Ragde over the past twenty years, we noticed that the patients, on average. were getting younger. Prostate cancer has, however, historically been called the disease for old men; if a man lives long enough, say into his 90's, there is a greater than 90% probability that he will have cancer of the prostate. But, it was also thought that such cancers didn't usually appear until men were well into their 60's or mid-70's. Even then, because prostate cancer has been seen as very slow growing, there was always the option to wait and watch, perhaps treating the (slow urination) symptoms while patients eventually succumbed of some other malady. Life spans for men, after all, is still mid-to late 70's, so taking a slow and deliberate approach to prostate cancer treatment selection seemed the right approach in a majority of cases.

In the last decade of the 20th century, however, the average age of prostate cancer patients declined (Southwest Oncology, 2001). In a study quoted by Dr. Schachter (Health World OnLine, 2001), careful pathological examinations of the prostate glands during the autopsies of men killed in accidents revealed some alarming statistics. According to Schachter, *"the study showed that the incidence of microscopic prostate cancer was 80% in men between the ages 70 and 80 years old, 40% in men between 50 and 60 years old, 34% in men between 40 and 50 years old, and 27% in men between 30 and 40 years old."* These are alarming numbers, even realizing that they refer to *microscopic* prostate cancer and not to *clinical* prostate cancer (which is diagnosed when a person is alive).

The Southwest College of Naturopathic Medicine, SCNM Newsletter (www.scnm.edu, Winter-2003 issue) also reported that a New York postmortem study found undiagnosed prostate cancer in men in their early twenties. So, the medical community at least realizes this is no longer just a disease that *only* older men get. With new diagnostics technology arriving every day, we are coming to realize that PC is a bigger risk to men than anyone ever thought possible---and younger men are seemingly at risk, too.

The autopsies used in the studies quoted were conducted for other reasons than to compile prostate information so that the conclusions drawn about cancer cells in the prostates of younger men are certainly unbiased. But they are startling and illuminating. What this says for the researchers who are trying to find out what causes the spontaneous emission of cancer cell growth in the prostate is, *such microscopic cancer cells may be present in a large segment of the male population* and isolating the trigger mechanism for onset is more crucial than thought, particularly if we are ever to eliminate or eradicate prostate cancer.

The idea that prostate cancer screening should begin in men at the age of 50 is supported by, among others, the American Cancer Society, NCCN, and the American Urological Association (UAU). Those organizations say that screening should occur annually because early detection of prostate cancer can lead to successful treatment. On the other hand, a federally funded 2002 study concluded that *"the risk of prostate cancer is so low for these men (*under age 50*), that checking once every two years, or even every five years, is enough to find cancer in time."* (__AP; May 21, 2002)

The study results were reviewed by one of its authors, University of Colorado professor E. D. Crawford at the Orlando American Society of Clinical Oncology (May 20, 2002), where he noted that, the recommendations for further testing should be based on PSA levels. He said the study concludes that where PSA readings are between zero and 1.0 ng per milliliter, a man can wait 5 years to have another test. If reading is between 1.0 and 2.0, a man can wait two years to have another test, and those whose readings are between 2 and 4.0 ng per milliliter should continue to have annual tests. *"If* (the study guidelines are*) followed,"* Dr. E. D. Crawford noted, *"(this) will mean much less testing for the majority of men..."*

It should be noted, however, that all of this, (*not* overtly highlighted in the study) was an attempt to reduce the **cost** of screening for prostate cancer, as noted in the fine print which said that, if the guidelines are followed, the number of PSA tests per year would be cut in half and a savings (to insurance companies?) of $500 Million to $1 Billion would be realized nationwide.

This study and its conclusions are obviously at odds with the statistics on incidence of prostate cancer. It may be an artifact of how the study was set up or, it may be 'creative statistics' being used to show a way to reduce medical costs. It was a "federally funded" study but little information is available on what agency sponsored it or for what reason the study was conducted. Common sense (and a look at 'creative statistics') would show, however, that reducing the number of PSA tests performed only reduces the number of 'potential' cancers detected. If you don't look for it, you won't find it so avoiding the $10 - $20 PSA lab cost in yearly physical exams (i.e. saving the insurance companies $50 to $100 over five annual exams) is likely to result in a much higher incidence of positive results in men 55 years of age. But, the percentage of those diagnosed men having *'confined'* prostate cancer at that point in their lives, will likely be fewer than if it had been screened (and detected) five years before. Is it worth it? Ask the man who follows this guideline *after* he finds out his prostate cancer is unconfined, what *he* thinks of his doctor's (and this study's) advice.

As a result of the data compiled for Edition 2.0 of this book, it is even more clear that PSA screens should begin even earlier than is currently recommended. Rather than age 50, as has been recommended by the ACS and other medical and oncology organizations, we believe the proper time to include PSA in annual physical exams is between the ages of 40 and 45. If there is a family history of prostate cancer, age 40 would be recommended and, where PSA results at that time were less than 1.0, perhaps screening every other year until age 50 would be the recommendation. Of course, if symptoms manifest themselves during the ages 40 to 50, more diagnostics are required. After age 50, the data suggest that *all* men should have an annual physical examination with *both* a DRE and PSA. Nothing in studies or the literature utilized in the research for this book changes that recommendation.

Again, its communication that is important. As noted before, most middle aged men haven't even thought about prostate health at the age of 40. And, yes, 40 is middle aged, like it or not! But making it through the 'second half' of your life, requires understanding what options are available (for such threats to your health as cancer). Therefore, making the information available and publicizing it to men early is just as important as publicizing breast cancer information to women at an early stage. We believe that men have the intelligence to take care of their own health by age 40 and that prostate cancer information is just as important to communicate to them as are the so called 'fitness' and 'workout' commercials aimed at the aging 'boomers every day in the media. Let's be sure we are communicating the *right* message: *'fit at 40 and beyond,'* should be our mantra. Prostate health should be a part of that mantra, also.

OTHER TREATMENTS AND STUDIES OF INTEREST

When the First Edition of this book went to press, a very promising vaccine was being developed by clinical researchers at Johns Hopkins. At the time, the FDA said..." it is 'promising' and they expected to approve it within a couple of years." Potentially, what a vaccine would mean would be that, like other childhood diseases which vaccines have eradicated, the vaccine could be administered at a young (yet-to-be-determined) age and, like polio, the world (i.e. *all* men!) could quit worrying about it.

(Note: Polio, in early 2012, is on the rebound in sub-tropic countries as this goes to press---so, even a vaccine must be delivered to be successful)

Unfortunately, the optimistic speculation has not lived up to the expectations of the Johns Hopkins researchers, so in the meantime, we must keep trying to find the cause (i.e. we still don't know why cancer starts in the first place) while spreading the word about the variety of successful treatments available, for the foreseeable future.

Also, as noted earlier in this chapter, in another study conducted at the University of Michigan Medical School in 2001/2002, researchers examined tumor cells taken from prostate cancer patients and found 55 genes that were more active in metastatic cells than in less-lethal cells. A gene called EZH2 showed that its activity increased as the disease progressed. And, patients who showed higher levels of the EZH2 protein were more likely to get the deadlier form of the disease.

Dr. A.M. Chinnaiyan, an assistant professor of pathology and a lead investigator in the study noted that,

> ***"...it suggests that this is a lethal biomarker, that portends aggressiveness... and, if a test can be developed, EZH2 protein levels could be used to decide which patients need aggressive treatment, including radiation and/or surgery."***

The study, published in the October 11, 2002 edition of Nature, also pointed out that many men over 60 years of age are receiving unnecessary surgery and other treatments for prostate cancer that is unlikely to spread...and that this new biomarker may be one answer for screening out those men who should have further treatment from those who should not. At this time, in 2012, however, the EZH2 screening tool may still be unavailable in most hospitals so it still remains to be seen where this research will lead.

COMMON TREATMENT OPTIONS TODAY: Radical Prostatectomy (Surgery)

As mentioned before, the most common treatment being recommended today for prostate cancer is radical prostatectomy (i.e. surgical removal of the prostate gland). Remember: it's not called, '**radical'** for nothing. For men who are older than 75 or 80, this may be a good option if certain conditions exist (assuming, once again, that the cancer is found to be confined to the prostate gland and enlargement of the gland is not correctable any other way). But, as noted before, for men older than 70 or 75, there may be good reason to just 'watch and wait' and see what other maladies become more important to your longevity---it probably isn't prostate cancer that will be your final downfall, if the cancer is confined to the capsule---so for this man, get on with living life and enjoy your retirement! For a 'younger' man, however, these questions are important unless:

Condition #1: Sex is no longer important or necessary in your life.

It's generally thought that men in their twilight years have little or no sex life. From studies and reports based on retirement communities in the southwestern U.S. (i.e. remember the sexy Sun City, Arizona residents caught having 'relations' outdoors in 2000?) this may be a false assumption. GP's and urologists know that healthy men over the age of 70 are likely to still be having sex at least once or twice a month, sometimes more frequently. Men between the ages of 50 and 70 are likely to have sex even more frequently, so, for a man of *any* age (not just 75 or older) who is diagnosed with prostate cancer and a radical prostatectomy is recommended, answering this question should be the first priority

Condition #2: Impotence will be almost certain but so will incontinence.

After a Radical Prostatectomy, incontinence occurs in 90% of all men for a period lasting from three months to forever. The severity of incontinence may range from total loss of control to partial loss of control (at each urination event). But, 40% to 50% of all men who have a radical prostatectomy have incontinence *forever*. Yes, they do have diapers now for adults, but is that what you really want to have happen? Think about it!

Condition #3: Radical Prostatectomy does not guarantee that cancer won't return later:
(...even though many urologists will say it is the only sure "treatment" that eliminates cancer)

For many reasons, removal of the prostate gland does not guarantee that cancer cells have not already migrated outside the prostate gland (i.e. it is unconfined) before surgery. One of the ways this happens, as discussed earlier, is during the biopsy. But, there are other reasons and most of them will never be discussed with the patient.

When a radical prostatectomy is performed, the layers of the gland are peeled away like the layers of an onion until only the outer "skin" is left attached to the various tissue that once held the gland in place. If cancer cells are present in this layer of skin, they are immediately available to migrate to other parts of the body. Thus, removal of the gland can still leave behind cancer cells that will grow to live another day in another place in the body. In fact, they may be in the groin area within days of the biopsy being performed. But, certainly they can be "spread" in the surgical process of radical prostatectomy. Even the surgeons will not discount that possibility, preferring instead to point to the "10 year survival" rates of 80+% of their patients. The question is, when you are under the age of 45 to 50, is ten years enough?

TWO PROCEDURES ARE COMMON: A Third Procedure Is 'Available'

According to doctors at the Mayo Clinic, two procedures are commonly available for a radical prostatectomy: retropubic and perineal surgery. In retropubic surgery, the gland is taken out through an incision in the lower abdomen that typically runs from just below the navel to about an inch above the penis. It's the most common form of prostate removal because lymph nodes surrounding the prostate can be removed and tested to make sure the cancer hasn't spread. Plus, the procedure gives the surgeon better access to the prostate, making it easier to save the nerve bundles that control erection (although, they may not always be undamaged).

Perineal surgery utilizes an incision made between the anus and the scrotal sac holding the testicles. This method generally involves less bleeding and heavier men recover sooner but, because the approach is much more difficult than retropubic surgery, it is much more difficult to locate and save the nerve bundles. Of course, lymph nodes are not accessible in this method and that is the reason this procedure is less commonly used.

Just announced in 2010, a third radical prostatectomy procedure is being pioneered at Mayo Clinic by Dr. Mitchell Humphreys at the Mayo Clinic Hospitals in Scottsdale, Arizona has developed a prostate surgical technique that is called Natural Orifice Transluminal Endoscopic Surgical Radical Prostatectomy, now referred to as NOTES RP. This is a procedure that builds on other "natural" techniques such as removing an appendix through a mouth or a gall bladder or kidneys via the vagina.

According to Dr. Humphreys, even though the 'procedure' may not be for the squeamish, it does have the advantage that it leaves little or no scarring and recovery time is reduced along with the risk of infection---which seems to go along with the trend to use robotic procedures in more and more surgical settings.

This procedure was actually developed while Humphries was interning at the Mayo in Rochester, Minnesota with two other urologists and the procedure is now being used exclusively at other Mayo hospitals. Special instruments were actually developed which allow the dissecting of the prostate gland and removal of the small dissected particles through the urethra. The prostate 'internal' tissues are then rejoined to the bladder with instruments that are also inserted through the urethra, thereby requiring no surgical opening as in a traditional radical prostatectomy procedure.

This is a relatively "new" procedure and the jury is still out on what benefits, other than the quicker recovery times and no scarring, are for this procedure. Obviously, no catheter is inserted (at least, not during the procedure; perhaps one is inserted post-operation?), but the comparison of long-term effectiveness as measured by how long a patient lives after the procedure is performed is still to be seen. This procedure has only been used for the past 2+ years on humans (men), so the numbers of successful surgeries utilizing this NOTES RP procedure are still accumulating.

One cautionary note to ask two questions about before embarking on this (or any other 'brand new technique' for prostate surgery), relates to the issue of how cancer cells might be allowed to spread outside the prostate gland itself. It was previously noted in this chapter that performing a simple biopsy carries with it the possibility or risk that cancer cells can be allowed to migrate down the needle-pathways during and following a biopsy. With this NOTES RP procedure, the fact that the prostate is actually 'dissected' and removed in very tiny pieces THROUGH the urethra, begs the question: are those prostate particles *which contain tiny cancer cells*, encapsulated so that they are totally isolated from the inside layers of the urethra or, are they allowed to 'touch' the inner walls of the urethra, which would propagate the migration of those tiny cancer cells into the urethra walls and further into the lymph system in the groin area?

Also, the actual reattachment of the bladder to (former) prostate tissues is already a potential source for cancer cells (post-surgery) migration. How does this *NOTES RP* procedure reduce the risk that those same pathways for cancer cell migration shouldn't be addressed with this procedure? It is possible that the Mayo specialists can explain that concern, if the question is addressed directly. Information was not available on either of these questions at the time this Edition 2.0 went to press.

Newer robotic procedures are being used now at most hospitals across the country. These robotic procedures are becoming more sophisticated and doctors who use them are becoming more skilled at their art, which allows the procedure to be done with less pain for the patient, less loss of blood and no scars. According to doctors at Scottsdale (Arizona) Shea Healthcare hospital (AZ Republic Supplement, 6/2/03), the daVinci Surgical System provides three-dimensional magnification not available with traditional laparoscopic equipment and utilizes 3 computerized robotic arms, one with a 3-D camera and the other two with precision surgical instruments. The pencil-sized arms are placed inside the patient through small incisions and are maneuvered by the surgeon who sits at a console a few feet from the operating table. This robotic procedure causes less discomfort and a return to normal activity more rapidly than a traditional laparoscopic prostatectomy procedure. More information on the promising daVinci surgical procedure is in Chapter Seven.

It is important to note, however, that success rates in preserving continence and erectile function appear to be similar between prostatectomies done with the daVinci method and those done through open surgery, although studies detailed in the Journal of Urology (Nov. '02) indicate that, in prospective studies, Robotic RP patients rarely have incontinence or erectile dysfunction longer than two years after surgery. So, while expectations for better outcomes may or may not be increased with the daVinci surgical procedures, the discomforts of the surgical process itself are much reduced.

It should be also noted that not every urologist/surgeon is trained on robotic systems so the availability of this procedure should cause the interested patient to seek out more than one opinion on what surgery (if any), and at which clinics experienced robotics surgeons reside. The answers you get, in part, may depend upon the experience of the surgeon you talk to so seek out more than one opinion even if you already have decided that robotic surgery is your best option;

you want to be sure you choose the most experienced prostate doctor manning the robotics controls.

So, for the man who understands the three conditions, it should be easier to make a decision to go ahead with a radical prostatectomy (or ***not***). But, for most men, this should be a _last_ choice. That is the reason for recommending getting second and third opinions before making a life-changing decision---no matter what your choice of treatment is---it is your quality of life afterwards that is important.

Even for the man who appears to have cancer cells outside the prostate gland, the choice for radical prostatectomy is still not definite. In fact, for the man in this situation, such surgery might be totally unnecessary, and working on finding and eliminating the cancer cells that have migrated outside the gland should be a first priority. (This is what is intended when surgeons administer hormone shots, or hormonal therapy, discussed later in Chapter Seven). Again, there are different options for the man in this circumstance and obtaining second and third opinions are absolutely essential.

Remember also, that even recognized treatment centers like the Mayo Clinic understand that radical prostatectomy patients have a nearly 30% reoccurrence rate (www.mayoclinic.com; 2001). Again, these kinds of statistics should send up red flags: explore all your options before deciding on prostate cancer (treatment) solutions.

OTHER OPTIONS: EXTERNAL BEAM RADIATION AND BRACHYTHERAPY

In a later chapter there is a discussion of cutting edge therapies now under development in Europe and the US. Those therapies may be an option for men, even today, under certain circumstances. However, the _proven_ therapies (i.e. those that are showing cure results of 80% to 97% (in men treated since the early-'90's) are called:

External Beam Radiation;

Brachytherapy (Radioactive Seed Implants);

Radical Prostatectomy.

These three treatments for prostate cancer are statistically about equal in their success at stopping cancer (for ten years). That is, all three of these treatments have been tracked in various studies and have been found to be about equally effective for men living ten years afterwards (or for men who died during that time of some other cause). In other words, for all practical purposes, choosing one or the other of the three treatments had the same results: cancer was 'cured' (i.e. 'cured' means the patients lived ten more years after treatment).

In a New England Journal of Medicine (NEJM) Case Study (2011-ONLINE), nationally recognized prostate cancer doctors at Massachusetts General Hospital reviewed the history of a 65 year old man who had been treated 6 years before with brachytherapy and had recently had urinary bleeding follow-up tests that were inconclusive (PSAs were <0.2 and the resected urethra tumor cells were negative for p63, PSA, prostate-specific acid phosphatase (PSAP), cytokeratin

(CK) 7, and thyroid transcription factor 1 (TTF-1) and positive for CDX2 and CK20). During the discussion that followed for the NEJM Morning Report, Dr. D Kauffman noted that,

> *"It is generally considered that surgery in all its forms (open prostatectomy, laparoscopic prostatectomy, robot-assisted radical prostatectomy) and radiation in all its forms (conformal external-beam radiation therapy, using either intensity-modulated radiation treatment or protons, and brachytherapy) are similarly effective for cancer control. The side-effect profiles differ for surgery and radiation, however. With surgery, incontinence and impotence are the main side effects. With radiation, impotence occurs with about the same frequency as with surgery, whereas incontinence is very uncommon. With radiation, bleeding from the rectum or bladder or both may occur and may persist for years."*

In further analysis by the Massa General team, Dr. Anthony Zietman noted that:

> *This man had a normal-size gland and most likely a very small tumor volume and was treated with brachytherapy--- brachytherapy, which means "close therapy," is a form of radiation treatment in which the radiation is locally released into a tumor from radioactive sources ("seeds") inserted directly into it. This is distinct from teletherapy ("distant therapy," more commonly known as external-beam irradiation), in which a radiation beam is directed into the body from an external source. Brachytherapy is an attractive choice for this patient, because high doses of radiation can be delivered exactly where they are required, with little or no irradiation of adjacent tissues. However, in the past, the use of brachytherapy was limited by factors such as the risk to caregivers from radium and radon sources,1 the requirement for an open procedure to insert the seeds, the inaccuracy of freehand seed insertion, and the advanced nature of most cancers at diagnosis.*
>
> *In recent years, a confluence of events has brought brachytherapy back into favor. First, PSA testing allows for the detection of cancers at an earlier stage, as in this patient, when cure is feasible with local treatment. Second, improvements in ultrasound technology and the transrectal probe allow better visualization of the prostate and permit transperineal source insertion under accurate image-guidance.*

If the "success rate" is about equal with the three treatment types, making a treatment selection is, at least in significant part, ***a quality-of-life-after-treatment-decision***---what quality of life do you want to have, after treatment? As explained in the discussion on Radical Prostatectomy earlier, side effects of that treatment are a *major* consideration.

If E-Beam treatments are conducted over several weeks, as is typically recommended (i.e. 5 to 7 weeks, E-Beam radiation 5 days out of seven each week), there is usually "burning" of sensitive tissues near and surrounding the prostate gland that last several months.* In this procedure, radiation is delivered by a beam from a large machine placed over the body. Unfortunately, these "external beams" do more than destroy cancerous cells; they can damage healthy tissue in the same area and that is why the first step in radiation therapy is to map out the areas in your body to receive radiation.

Three-dimensional scans show the location of the prostate and surrounding organs, then computer imaging software allows a radiation therapist to rotate the picture in any direction to find the best angles to direct the beams. For External Beam Radiation, also called 'E-Beam,' side effects are related to the amount and number of E-Beam treatments the patient undergoes. In addition, side effects also may be related to the location of the tumor(s) in the prostate gland and the pathway the E-Beam travels to reach the tumor(s).

In some cases, for example, where tumor(s) are near the inside surface of the gland and in close proximity to the anus, the E-Beam actually 'radiates' or burns areas around the sensitive anus tissue as it irradiates the cancer cells inside the prostate gland. This patient will suffer pain and discomfort in the groin and anus area for weeks or even months afterwards. Doctors recommending this treatment are beginning to explore different treatment schemes now in an effort to minimize this after effect but the man choosing this therapy should expect several weeks or even months of after-effects.

It is also true that oncology/radiologists are using E Beam treatments before Brachytherapy, just to ensure that cancer cells that might have migrated outside the prostate gland (but remain in the general vacinity) are destroyed before radiation 'seeds' are implanted. This might involve only 2 or 3 E Beam treatments of a minute each that will usually not result in side effects that full E Beam treatment promote, although tumors located at or near the prostate surface might cause E Beam burning to the soft tissues, as noted before.

The Mayo Clinic (www.mayoclinic.com) notes that sexual impotence occurs in 30% to 50% of men treated with external beam radiation, that conclusion is not substantiated in other studies. Incontinence, however, is rare in E Beam patients.

> ***Note:** Two men interviewed for this Edition 2.0 had only two E-Beam treatments, (instead of the normal twenty to forty treatments over 4-6 weeks), just prior to getting the radioactive seed implants and a year later, both men had bleeding from radiation 'burns' on the inside of their colon where the E Beam passed through tissue surrounding the prostate.
>
> A third patient interviewed nearly 2 years after undergoing 5 weeks of E-Beam treatments, 35 treatments, followed by brachytherapy, continued to experience severe pain and bleeding in the colon and rectum accompanied by intermittent incontinence and some sexual dysfunction. Two years later, this man began to experience rising PSA scores and more bleeding. Ultimately, this man died seven years after being treated for prostate cancer with External Beam treatment.

BRACHYTHERAPY

The other type of radiation therapy that has become more and more popular is brachytherapy, or otherwise known as radioactive seed placement. In this treatment, ultrasound-guided needles are used to inject rice-grain sized radioactive "seeds" into the prostate around the tumors. These 'seeds,' either made up of iodine 150, palladium, or strontium, contain just enough radiation (i.e. about twice the dose of the E Beam) that the tumors are bombarded (for months after treatment) but healthy surrounding tissues are not affected.

The procedure is conducted in an operating room on an out-patient basis and takes about 90 minutes. Just as with surgery, the patient is anesthesized and needles containing the 'seeds' are inserted through the parineam and into the prostate around the tumor(s) that were identified previously in an ultrasound exam. In the recovery room after the implants are finished, the catheter is removed and the patient goes home, sometimes resuming a regular schedule the next day after treatment.

Because the procedure for inserting the radioactive seeds into the prostate gland is similar to the biopsy procedure, scar tissue will be gradually formed around the insertion pathways inside the gland. For the immediate 48 hours following the brachytherapy procedure, the urination of blood and a stinging sensation occurs throughout the length of the penis with each urination event. The blood in the urine eventually subsides, although it may persist for as much as a week or two. But, the stinging sensation ebbs and flows throughout the penis and into the bladder for weeks or months after the procedure. (Of all the after-effects, patients interviewed for this research said this 'burning' sensation and its variations were the most annoying).

Because the prostate gland provides the 'pump' and seminal fluid for ejaculation of the sperm in male orgasim, the first few times after treatment that a man has sex, the fluid will be bloody. Again, as with urination, this blood content diminishes over the first few weeks after treatment until no trace is seen. In most men, even though there is a fairly great amount of blood in the seminal ejaculation the first few times, there is very little pain and sex *should* be resumed almost without concern in a very short time span after the implant procedure.(*)

> *(**Note:** Dr. Grado was asked about how soon sex should be resumed after brachytherapy surgery and he replied, *"we prefer that patients wait until after they have been discharged from the hospital!"*)

The emphasis on '*should*' be resumed is intentional: in order to ensure that the prostate gland still functions properly, it is recommended that frequent sex is preferable to infrequent. Ejaculation helps to keep the prostate gland functioning while the scar tissue is building and it is thought that it will function better and longer into the future, if sex and ejaculation is resumed soon after treatment.

As noted before, one thing that all men who have had brachytherapy experience is the continued 'burning' sensation throughout the entire length of the penis and up into the urethra, whenever urinating. This is a 'sensation' that can only be understood by men who have experienced it but, suffice it to say, it manifests itself in the head of the penis sometimes, and sometimes throughout the length of the penis (feeling like it goes all the way back up into the bladder!). The sensation, usually very strong in the first days and weeks after treatment, varies in intensity over time, and lasts (in some men) a year or more.

The 'flow' of urine also varies in the brachytherapy patient. In the early weeks after brachytherapy, urine flow will be difficult sometimes, especially at night after sleep has induced a relaxed state to the bladder and urethra. Prescription medication can relieve these symptoms but will still be required in most men for months following the procedure.

One thing is for certain, while these side effects are sometimes painful and generally annoying, they do diminish over time. Thus, use of brachytherapy as a treatment of choice to eliminate cancer cells in the prostate gland should be considered to have the *least* side effects of concern (of the three most common treatments reviewed in this text) for long term health and quality of life.

Dr. David Beyer, an MD/Brachytherapist who pioneered seed implantation in the late 1980's at Scottsdale (Arizona) Healthcare noted in a supplement to the Arizona Republic in June of 2003, that *"...brachytherapy has several advantages to surgery or external radiation, (such as):*

* Fewer side effects than other treatments;

* Is less invasive than major surgery;

* Is less damaging to surrounding tissue;

* Has been proven effective against cancer (in the Prostate Gland).

Dr. Beyer noted that,

> ***"...we have long term follow-up data (now)"*** and ***"the chance of patients being cured are as good (with brachytherapy) as with any other treatment method."***

All that was based on data and experience with brachytherapy in the years prior to 2003 and the technology and skillful application of seed implants has only gotten better since then. Thus, the diagnosed patient should now find that this therapy may be a first choice when confronted with decisions about which therapy should be selected for treatment.

HORMONAL THERAPY

A discussion of treatment therapies would be incomplete without discussing Hormonal (Depravation) Therapy which is most certainly a well-established form of treatment for various and specific stages of prostate cancer. According to the Prostate Institute of America web site (July, 2003), the historical treatment of choice was to conduct a bilateral orchietctomy (removal of the testicles) to reduce or eliminate the male hormone, called androgen, production which is responsible for tumor growth.

This may seem a radical step to take but, for some patients whose cancer has spread outside the prostate capsule, it is/was a lifesaver. Recently, combination androgen ablation therapy was introduced and commercially available to maximize androgen blockade. Here's how this type of therapy works: There are two major organs in the human body that excrete male hormone. The major source is testicles and the second source is the adrenal glands. Types of drugs specifically for blocking the hormones excreted by the testicles are called LHRH agonists, such as Lupron or Zoladex. Flutamide or Casodex are the primary drugs used for adrenal gland hormone blockades.

However, there are some known complications on these drugs. Some experience hot flashes, diarrhea, insomnia, liver function damage and untold effects on the cardiovascular system and some men experience noticeable enlargement of the breast areas. But, for men in these circumstances, there are few treatment choices and strict supervision of hormonal deprivation therapy by a specialized physician is vital.

The Prostate Institute of America notes that combination androgen ablation therapy can be used as a primary form of treatment if someone has advanced cancer and it most likely will work but effective treatment results show no cancer growth for 3 to 5 years, then usually tumor growth starts again. Thus, it is important to know the pros and cons before choosing this treatment and understand how progress should be carefully monitored.

The Institute also notes on its website that "the major problem of prostate cancer treatment is under-estimation of the disease, or thinking it's understaged." In studies cited, they note that on the basis of their radical surgery (prostatectomy) experiences, approximately 50% of all cancers thought to be localized in the prostate have actually escaped out of the prostate capsule. (Note: they do not say or suggest when cancer cells might have migrated outside the capsule; see Chapter Three discussion of biopsy and brachytherapy cell migration).

The Institute notes that,

> ***"...since androgen blockade therapy can decrease the size of the tumor and the size of the prostate itself, the chances of an unexpected tumor extension outside of prostate at the time of surgery is minimized (downstaged)."***

It is unclear if the Institute made this observation to further enhance the desirability of seeking a prostatectomy as the treatment of choice or if the observation was for information purposes.

Whatever the reasons, selection of hormonal therapy (with or without combining it with another treatment) should be considered only in cases where the tumors are thought to have spread outside the prostate capsule. For this reason, most statistics on this type of therapy have come from men over the age of their late 70's and may have to be reevaluated for men in their younger 50's to early 70's.

FINASTERIDE TRIALS: BPH vs Cancer Risk

In June of 2003, the National Cancer Institute published results of studies in the the New England Journal of Medicine about the (then) new drug, Finasteride. At that time, it looked like a potential 'silver bullet' might have been found, at least for men who suffered with BPH, in reducing their risk of contracting prostate cancer. The study utilized the BPH-reduction drug, finasteride, in a study at University of Texas Health Sciences Center in San Antonio, where 18,000 men over the age of 60, were tracked for more than seven years and what they wanted to know was, did the administration of finasteride reduce the risk that men who suffered BPH would get cancer.

The most popular use for finasteride, or Proscar as it is named on the prescription market, although in significantly less dosage than was administered in this study, is for baldness prevention. It is also used for BPH sufferers, and the study utilized similar dosage in this study as that used for the purpose of reducing the symptoms of prostate gland enlargement.

Dr. Ian Thompson was the Principle Investigator on the study and he noted that Proscar alters levels of the male hormone, DHT, a testosterone relative. It has already been determined that men with naturally low levels of DHT have less prostate cancer and that Black (American) men who generally have a very high risk of prostate cancer, have high DHT levels, also. In this study, researchers tested whether reducing DHT could prevent cancer and what they found was that men who took the drug every day for seven years reduced the risk of prostate cancer by 25 percent (15 fewer cancers in 1,000 men) as measured against the men in the study who were administered a placebo over the same period.

But, just in case this is the only article you might have read on the wonders of Finasteride, you should also know that other studies are showing that it may not be a silver bullet for men who face a decision of getting a biopsy (or not). In a Journal of New England Medicine editorial, (April, 2010), Dr. James Walsh cites studies being conducted in Finland that seems to show that use of hormone treatment may lead to a false sense of well-being. He concludes with this:

What advice should we be giving our patients (about long term results)?

> Dr. Walsh: "Dutasteride and finasteride do not prevent prostate
> cancer but merely temporarily shrink tumors
> that have a low potential for being lethal, and
> they do not reduce the risk of a positive biopsy
> in patients who have an elevated PSA level (corrected
> for the effect of the drug) or an abnormal
> digital rectal examination. Furthermore, the use
> of these drugs for *prevention* (emphasis added) may be somewhat
> risky. Because PSA levels are suppressed, men may
> have a false sense of security, and if prostate cancer
> ever develops, the diagnosis may be delayed
> until they have high-grade disease that may be difficult
> to cure."
>
> Walsh, NEJM 362;13 nejm.org April 1, 2010

Other Hormone-Deprivation Drugs: Stop Cancer in its Tracks!

For men who already know they have prostate cancer and have found their cancer has metastasized and who are in need of other life-extending treatments, the FDA approved the drug Jevtana, made by French drug maker, Sanofi-Aventis, for treating prostate cancer that does not respond to hormone-deprivation treatments or to docetaxel (the drug used most commonly to fight prostate tumors), for advanced cancer patients. In a 2009 study, Jevatana prolonged survival for those patients by 10 weeks and the hope is, for patients who are not as sick that administering Jevtana may extend survival even longer.

FDA's Office of Oncology Drug Products is quoted as saying..."patients have therapeutic options in this disease setting..." so allowing the use of this newly available drug will offer hope to a small percentage of men who are in this extreme situation.

The FDA felt compelled to act on this earlier than they had planned so that this treatment therapy could be used right away in clinical trials across the country.

UPSIDE vs. DOWNSIDE

While the news that prostate cancer might be prevented, and there might someday be a pill that every man could take to drive down the risk of having cancer later on, appears to be supported by the results of this study, there are some downside cautions to consider. The doctors conducting the study noted that Proscar (finastride) can cause sexual "problems" and, although not confirmed precisely by the study, the percentage of those men who did have prostate cancer during the study, appeared to have slightly more aggressive tumors than would have been expected in the normal population.

It should be noted that men in this prevention study had biopsies of their prostate glands, regardless of what their PSA levels were, in order to confirm tumors were present. Interestingly, researchers diagnosed prostate cancer in four times more placebo patients than expected in the normal population (non-trial-participants). Most tumors discovered were small, early-stage tumors which would not have triggered a biopsy under normal examination conditions.

The fact that the rate was four times higher than expected in the placebo group is actually consistent with the study noted earlier in this text (Chapter One) where the autopsies showed a very high presence of cancer tumors in prostates of men of all ages. But, this study's researchers made no comment about the significance of the findings in that regard.

What they did conclude is that the study gives hope that, one day, a vaccine or pill may be found that will be able to prevent prostate cancer on-set, much like the polio and small pox vaccines have accomplished for those diseases. Right now, however, they caution that the upside and downside of Finasteride therapy (as a prevention therapy) needs to be weighed by each individual who contemplates using it in the hope of preventing prostate cancer from occurring. Since the study didn't test whether taking the drug helped men live longer, American Cancer Society's Dr. Herman Kattlove predicted that there will be a huge debate about its usefulness.

It is interesting that there are continuing studies utilizing hormonal therapy drugs being conducted which are showing promise, some of which are looking at drugs that are being used to treat BPH, which seem to be showing that these drugs at least, can slow down the growth of cancer cells in the prostate gland. In January of 2011, preliminary results of a 3+ year study conducted at the Princess Margaret Hospital in Toronto, Canada where 300 men with low-risk cancer (i.e. are these 'insignificant' in previous studies?), confirmed by biopsies were given BPH drugs Avodart (dutasteride) or Proscar (finastride), to determine if they might also be effective in preventing the "*progression*" of prostate cancer tumors---slowing their growth down thereby allowing more time for a more thorough investigation into which treatment therapy ultimately would be the best choice.

The diagnosed men were given daily Avodart <u>or</u> placebo pills and biopsied one and a half to three years later. Results were that 38% of men taking Avodart and 49% of men on the placebo got worse while the final biopsies showed no signs of cancer in 36% of men on Avodart versus 23% of men on the placebos. Doctors who participated in the studies say that this last result shows how tin many of these cancers were to start with and that they just could not be found in the final biopsies---they don't think Avodart can cure cancers, but they do think it slows down the progression---but it is still unclear what the real results of this clinical trial means for men who are diagnosed with PC.

The results for the Proscar drug in these clinical trials were unavailable as this Edition 2.0 went to press but, suffice it to say, these studies show promise for slowing down prostate cancer's progression but for the man who is looking for a silver bullet---the "pill" that will cure PC---these study results are not the answer. That is pretty much in agreement with LA Cedars-Sinai Medical Center leading prostate cancer specialist Dr. Howard Sandler had to say, when asked about these preliminary findings: "(Avodart) is not likely a cure for PC but it does seem to suppress it."

The fact that one of the sponsors of the study was Avodart maker, GlaxoSmithKline should only be a concern if subsequent studies that are being conducted, fail to replicate the results of these studies. It remains to be seen what the Proscar study results are, but if they prove to be equally optimistic about their application to low-risk (insignificant cancers?) PC sufferers, it will certainly lead to more studies at clinics throughout the U.S. and something that offers hope for finding that long-sought "silver bullet" that might make PC, like polio and small pox, a thing of the past.

There is more in the Chapter Five about hormonal therapies, but suffice it to say, for our purposes in this Edition 2.0, all these studies are positive indicators that, eventually, it may be possible to have a pill that can be taken early on to prevent the onset of cancer that is the second leading cancer that causes men to die today. But, no 'silver bullet' is available today, so watching the progress in the medical community is our only option.

SUMMARY

Being diagnosed with a prostate <u>*problem*</u> doesn't automatically mean prostate <u>*cancer*</u>: it really means that a journey into uncharted medical territory is about to be undertaken. What direction is chosen is individual circumstance-driven: each man needs to begin the journey with the goal of living a healthy life, no matter what the diagnosis shows. In order to take the right steps toward that goal, information needs to be obtained and opinions of medical professionals sought that will lead to a successful outcome. If cancer is diagnosed in this journey, treatment options are available which can have a high probability of meeting the goal expectations.

A 2002 AARP magazine article, <u>*My Generation*</u> (July-August 2002) highlighted the journey taken by author/writer Hal Ackerman when he learned during a routine physical that he had prostate cancer. It is one man's view, very well written and clearly descriptive, of the ebb and flow of emotions a man feels as he goes through the process of dealing with prostate cancer. Ackerman's ability to paint his emotions in graphic color that can easily be understood are outstanding and we recommend the article to anyone with an interest in prostate cancer. His description of getting the biopsy results, while not necessarily accurate, deals head-on with the feelings those dreaded words evoke:

'"...you've got cancer...!'"

These are the words no one ever expects to hear and, thus, how one deals with those results becomes the foundation for making treatment choices based on many, many opinions by the medical community. It is highly recommended reading! For example, Ackerman retained his sense of humor, even though there are serious issues to debate.

On Radical Prostatectomy (surgical removal of the prostate gland), Ackerman quipped:

> ***'...given the proximity of the prostate to the male anatomy, you're cutting past a lot of delicate apparatus here. All the plumbing and hydraulics..'. ..."Oh, sorry. Did you want those balls??"*** **(Makes radiation sound a lot more enticing...) p 16**

In another case discussed in the Arizona Republic (2003), Dwight Schaeffer was 59 when he was diagnosed with prostate cancer at the Mayo Clinic during a routine physical exam. He was otherwise healthy and had no symptoms. A biopsy revealed that his was a fast-growing cancer so, after discussion with the urologist, talked to the radiologist who helped him decide on Electron Beam Therapy. This was more than a decade ago, when most non-surgical procedures were in their infancy but Dwight didn't like the surgery statistics, saying, "it was a risk but it was the right decision."

Dwight, however wasn't content to sit down and retire. He'd been an active working adult and wanted to continue running for his own well being and mental therapy. After his therapy, the 71 year-old was running 40 to 50 miles a week, became a USA Master's All-American in the 1500 meters for his age group (six minutes, 19 seconds) and credited "running for being a big part of the equation that led to my recovery...as part of a holistic approach to cancer management." The Mayo Clinic," he says, "has always supported his efforts in that regard." It is a footnote here, that I could not find information about Dwight while preparing this edition but it would be interesting to find out if Dwight is still going strong as he begins the second decade of the new millennium---we can only presume he is!

After his treatment, at age 60, after the E Beam treatment was doing its job, he went back to school and became a neuromuscular therapist, then moved to Arizona. He recommends,

> ***"...as a prostate patient, becoming an informed patient, doing your research on your condition verses the options for treatment, and incorporating a holistic approach into your treatment regimen that includes diet and exercise"***

Dwight's experience (and outcomes) were much different than the patient we interviewed in the note earlier proving, once again, it is important to find the *best* treatment for the circumstances a person is in, and, more importantly, spending the time to find the *best* doctor/clinic to conduct the treatment. It is apparent that, once a treatment decision has been made, it is important to find the best "applications-doctor" to do the treatment. The one with the *most* experience who has perfected the "art" of treatment, is the place you want to put your trust in.

Thus, its like choosing an artist to paint your portrait: The final result will be most positive if you find the "artist" who can do the work properly. The analogy holds for brachytherapy, external beam, or radical prostatectomy: Do your homework; seek more than one or two opinions, then make your choice with confidence.

OTHER BOOKS ABOUT PC WORTH READING

It was noted in the First Edition that there are very few books published by the popular press on Prostate Cancer, for a variety of reasons. Most books written on the subject are personal experiences, written much like a diary of events that took place when the diagnosis was positive. Most publishing houses are not interested in books, even in life and death chronicles about cancer, unless they are written by celebrities or recognized medical professionals. Thus, the *Primer First Edition* was not published by a big-name publisher because it was not a big seller that made either the author or the publisher, any money. That's understandable and, even, acceptable to the authors, as long as whoever does publish it ensures that it gets into the right people's hands: doctors, hospitals, and (most important), men and women/partners who love them and who need to learn about prostate health and options for treatment.

There are two books, however, that are highly recommended that fall in the category of "personal experiences" of their authors but, which have lots of information about prostate health within their pages. Both are books that are published by internet companies (1stbooks.com) and are available digitally or in hard copy. A brief description follows later in this chapter **(*)**.

A third book that is highly recommended was published by the American Cancer Society (ACS) in 1996 through Random House, Inc., and is titled simply: ***PROSTATE CANCER, What Every Man – and His Family – Needs to Know***. It is an excellent book, written and edited by a team of doctors (D.G. Bostwick, G.T. MacLennan, and T.R. Larson), with input from many more in various clinics and medical treatment facilities across the U.S. (including, Dr. Gordon Grado, at that time head of Radiology at Mayo Clinic/Scottsdale, quoted elsewhere in this Edition 2.0. It is an excellent book because of its descriptions, if not its current relevance to prostate cancer today (i.e. much of the technology and treatment was still in its infancy in 1996), all these years after it was written.

The ACS book is highly recommended, with the caveat that a significant amount of it is out-dated. But, it is very well-written explanations of procedures and anatomical descriptions (which are not out-dated). It has a lot of those pictures and graphs and charts that are intentionally missing from this Edition 2.0 and all those things are located in this one excellently written source. Also, it is still available from the American Cancer Society and perhaps booksellers on the Web like Amazon.com. It's just too bad that no one at the ACS has edited or updated the 1996 materials in a version that more accurately reflects the current state of the art for prostate cancer treatment options.

(*)TWO BOOKS OF PERSONAL EXPERIENCES

PROSTATE CANCER BATTLE: IT'S STRICTLY YOUR DECISION is written by Professor Michael O'Hara and was published by 1st Books in 2001. It has not yet become a runaway best seller (and, it probably never will) but page for page, it has more good information and charts and diagrams than most doctor's offices. And, like this 2nd Edition (2.0) its all about providing options and written by a prostate cancer survivor with straight talk about taking control of your life.

In fact, Professor O'Hara might have provided more information than most men would want to look at. He has included copies of his PSA tests, biopsy results, MRI scans and a lot of actual written communications from his own journey that are highly enlightening. The cost of his book from the internet site is under five bucks so for a broad perspective, you can not beat Professor O'Hara's 225 pages of insight.

Interestingly, Professor O'Hara chose (Iodine) radiation seed treatment and in a post-script at the back of his book, he had this to say:

> ***"In retrospect, the only thing that would have made my road less pressured and the specific decision-making process smoother would have been to have had immediate access to a book on prostate cancer like this one (his book). Then, when first appraised by my HMO physician that I had flunked my prostate biopsy, I would have been prepared to deal with the dilemma with a great deal less emotion and frustration." (pp 219)***

DROP YOUR DRAWERS: Excellent Advice!

The second text that is also published by ***1st Books***, is available in both digital and hard copy, written by Dr. Rupert Wentworth, titled ***CAUGHT WITH MY PANTS DOWN (2002)*** is "about Prostate Cancer, Metastatic Prostate Cancer, and more." It is highly recommended reading because it illustrates what can happen when the chosen treatment is ineffective in stopping the spread of prostate cancer.

In particular, Dr. Wentworth went to one of the most prestigeous medical clinics in America and had a radical prostatectomy performed that, he presumed, cured his cancer. Five years later, in 2000, his cancer metasticized in other parts of his body and he commenced a journey that is, today, an ongoing struggle to stay alive and maintain a good quality of life in the process.

Both these books are personal journeys that echo what this Edition 2.0 is about: the more information a man can get about prostate treatment options, the better he will be able to reduce the risk factors and choose a successful treatment. We highly recommend both the Wentworth and O'Hara books, together with the ACS book for a complete understanding of prostate cancer. With those three books, plus this text and access to the internet sites recommended here, you have the most up-to-date decision-making tools available at this point in time (2010) on prostate cancer.

FACING CHOICES: Get More Opinions

Just as in our discussion earlier in this chapter, and in the books recommended above, Wentworth, O'Hara, Ackerman, and Schaeffer were all faced with treatment choices. And, while there may be fewer high-percentage treatment types than six or eight that are candidates, the three *proven* prostate cancer-killer therapies with the highest probability of success are Radical Prostatectomy, External Beam Radiation (E-Beam), and Brachytherapy. Each therapy has its advantages and disadvantages so the choice a man makes depends on his own individual (physical) situation. The good news, however, is that information is more and more available on how to make choices and your continued best health options are dependent on acquiring and using that information.

A THIRD BOOK FROM THE NATIONAL PROSTATE CANCER COALITION

Normally, I would not recommend books or texts which I have not reviewed but, the National Prostate Cancer Coalition in Washington, D.C. has a lot of good advice and a web site (www.pcacoalition.org) where they regularly update prostate cancer information and, they have a book available that is a bit of a different perspective that we recommend checking out. The book is written by the wife of a gentleman that NPCA says is the "nation's leading lay expert on prostate cancer." (Their words, not ours)

The reason I recommend this book is because it is written by a diagnosed man's wife and, therefore, offers advise and words of encouragement to other wives and *significant other's* going through the prostate cancer experience with their partners which is a point of view no other written materials seems to take. The author, (wife) Desiree Lyon Howe is also a board member of the NPCC and that probably has something to do with their endorsement of her book but it is worth checking out, especially for the "partners" of men diagnosed with this disease.

HUNDREDS OF MORE "PERSONAL" WRITINGS

As noted earlier, there are hundreds of articles and papers written by diagnosed men, appearing in magazines and medical references. The few we have chosen to mention here are, however, ones we considered to be the best range of information for the newly diagnosed man that needs to gather as much information as possible in as short a time as possible. Urologists and prostate cancer specialists will also have a lot of literature and reference materials but, just as with the advice to seek out second and third opinions on your specific problem, it is recommended that you seek out as many different books, magazines articles and sources of printed materials on the problem also, as there are literally hundreds of different ways to look at prostate cancer; your specific physical situation requires that you find the right treatment (application) for ***YOU***.

And, while you will find differing opinions and sometimes conflicting interpretations of the same data, you owe it to yourself (and your significant other) to sift and sort the information and decide what ***YOU*** need to do for your own peace of mind; not your doctors! S/he will not be the one living with the consequences of the treatment you choose, so be diligent and open-minded. And, above all else, ask questions and be persistent. Its ***YOUR*** life!

"IF YOU HAVE BEEN DIAGNOSED WITH CANCER (ANY CANCER... NOT *ONLY* PROSTATE CANCER), YOU ABSOLUTELY *MUST* SEEK MORE THAN ONE MEDICAL OPINION ABOUT YOUR TREATMENT OPTIONS! AND, YOU ABSOLUTELY *MUST* SEEK OPINIONS FROM DIFFERENT TREATMENT SPECIALISTS: SURGERY, RADIATION, CRYOGENICS, ROBOTICS SURGERY; ETC."

CHAPTER THREE

What you'll learn about in this chapter...

When is 'no treatment' the best option?

What urologists know or do not know (or tell)

What oncologists know or do not know (or tell)

Where to find reliable information

Second and Third Opinions: Whom do you trust?

INTRODUCTION

There is so much misinformation about Prostate Cancer in the media these days that it is no wonder men become confused when they are first diagnosed; where do you turn for advice you can trust? Lately, there have been an increasing number of reports that prostate cancer is being over-diagnosed. Imagine how that information makes you feel when you are not only looking for your best treatment options but thinking that maybe, you are one of those who shouldn't have even gotten a biopsy to begin with!

The gold standard test for prostate cancer is the PSA (Prostate-Specific Antigen) blood test that most likely was the 'indicator' that sent you to get a biopsy, and now, the University of Arizona professor of immunology and pathology, Dr. Richard Ablin, who actually discovered the PSA test--- has been quoted in a March 2010 editorial in the New York Times as saying that (PSA) testing has become a *'profit-driven public health disaster...'* that is costing the public $3 Billion a year...and leads to *OVER*-diagnosing prostate cancer. But, its driving the costs ever higher without appreciably increasing the accuracy of results that will make the treat or not-to-treat decision easier.

It is bad enough that journalists have little understanding about prostate cancer studies that they summarize in the media without having the very doctor who devised the best and most accurate blood test procedure that has led thousands of men to have biopsies, now confuses us even more by saying that...basically, ..."the PSA screening isn't very definitive...(whatever that means)..."...it can not distinguish between the two types of prostate cancer; the one that will kill you and the one that won't." It doesn't help that he tried to clarify by saying that 'other causes for fluctuating or high PSA numbers, like an infection or even a recent ingestion of ibuprofen, might be the reason (that PSA results were high); when the biopsy results are positive, the PSA was the indicator that led to the biopsy being performed so how can that be a bad thing?

E Magazine (Sep/Oct 2010) asks, "what's a guy to do?" They point out that the 'fear of dying' factor weighs heavily on a PSA decision and, typically, men are afraid NOT TO get a biopsy, even if their doctor's advise them to 'wait and watch'---this, then, according to Ablin, leads to over-diagnosis which doesn't then show whether the cancer (if diagnosed in the biopsy) is the "type that will likely kill or if it is the less aggressive type and should be left alone." But, that's never been the question that PSA results intended to answer. PSA is an indicator, and what ever that means should be a joint collaboration between the doctor and patient: wait and watch? Get a biopsy? Return in three months and get a new PSA? Those are the questions/answers that PSA screening are for, not for deciding which treatment (or not) should be undertaken.

After A Positive Biopsy Result

If you look at Dr. Ablin's admonishment, you can see that a positive outcome (i.e. a biopsy which shows cancer cells are present), does not mean that doctors can tell for sure if the cancer is (in his words) ...*"the type that will kill you or the type that won't."* But, the fact that cancer was detected at all likely would not have been the case even a decade ago, *without* the PSA screening tool, so at least there is a chance that the early detection has allowed treatment decisions to be a matter of choice, rather than looking at advanced stage cancers allow only limited treatment options.

It is commonly stated in articles and literature that prostate cancer is ***usually*** a very slow growing type of cancer. (emphasis on ***usually***) But, if you are diagnosed with prostate cancer, what does that mean? Do you have *years* to deal with it? Do you have *months*? Or, should you be dealing with it as soon as possible, even though it may be slow growing --- it could still be dangerous so shouldn't you do something as quickly as possible?

The answer to these questions, at least with today's medical knowledge of the subject is, **"it depends."** There are so many variables to consider when trying to determine what the time frame is for taking a treatment action that it is difficult to give a check sheet of options and a time line that meets every individual's situation.

Since the First Edition of this Primer was published, however, feedback from many men who were treated, and several who were not (i.e. those who chose to 'watch and wait' for some period following the biopsy), there is one variable that seems to be clear: for men who are older than 75, depending upon the Gleason score (*aggressivness* of the tumor(s), it is highly likely that watching and waiting is the least risk alternative to choosing a treatment---if the cancer is not (numerically) thought to be aggressive---it is far more likely that NO treatment will be the BEST treatment because a man in his early 70's will likely outlive the cancer and die of some other cause ten, fifteen or even 20-plus years in the future.

So, if you are older than 75 and your Gleason scores are 7 or less, *forget about it!!* Live the good life! Have a lot of sex and exercise that prostate gland; you earned it!

SECOND AND THIRD OPINIONS: ABSOLUTELY, *POSITIVELY*, REQUIRED!

The American Association of Retired People (AARP) monthly newsletter/bulletin in February, 2003 reported on the importance of getting second and third opinions for critical diagnosis. In the article, several cancer experts and clinical studies were quoted, one specifically relevant for prostate cancer: Professor Jerome Groopman, M.D. at the Medical School at Harvard University has even written a book on the importance of second opinions (Second Opinions, Penquin USA, 2001). He quotes Ernest Rosenbaum, M.D. who is in Clinical medicine at Stanford University who says,

> ***"...the question is not why you should get a second opinion but why would you not? There is no scientific downside."***

And, further, Groopman and Rosenbaum point out that most doctors *encourage* patients to seek out a second opinion, because they need to feel comfortable with their own diagnostics. Groopman notes that doctors who do not welcome a second opinion should serve as a red flag; something is wrong here.

Dr. Groopman notes,

> ***"...if your father had prostate cancer, he was probably told it had to be removed surgically and that was that. Today, a biopsy determines the stage of the cancer—and the recommended treatment can absolutely change as a result of subtle differences that may only be detected through a second opinion."***

That's good advice, and comes from years of diagnosing and treating varying types of cancer. Dr Groopman and Dr. Rosenblum, who chairs the Department of Pathology at Memorial Sloan-Kettering Cancer Center in New York City have been analyzing tumors for a combined total of more than 50 years. They point out that,

> ***"...analyzing even the rarest tumors is second nature to a pathologist in a specialized referral center, because we look at so many cases."***

Further, the technology in medicine diagnostics is changing so fast that (prostate) cancer solutions and treatment options are increasing at an exponential rate. The AARP article lists ways to get the most from a second opinion:

GETTING THE MOST FROM SECOND (AND THIRD) OPINIONS

(from Stanford University's Dr. Rosenbaum):

*Tell your doctor you want another review *and* enlist his help. "It's a terrible mistake to go behind your doctors back for a second opinion because you're afraid he'll be mad at you."

*Take notes during the second opinion interview, or even better, tape it, even if you're accompanied by a relative or friend. This lets you review the information at your own pace.

*If your health plan won't cover a second opinion, pay for one yourself if at all possible. (After all, it may be your life that hangs in the balance)

*Use organizations such as the American Heart Association, the American Cancer Society and the National Cancer Institute for information and referral sources. The Richard and Annette Bloch Cancer Foundation (www.blastcancer.org) offers a list of major cancer referral centers throughout the country.

*Approach second (and third) opinions on the Internet with extreme caution. Thousands of websites claim to offer opinions by qualified doctors, and it's difficult to detect the quacks.

*If your first and second doctors don't agree, get a third opinion (or more!). Medicare and many private health plans pay.

(Web sites you need to know and phone numbers where you can contact the experts: *American Heart Association*, www.americanheart.org or Ph (800)-242-8721; the *American Cancer Society*, www.cancer.org or (800)-227-2345; the *National Cancer Institute*, (www.nci.nih).

YOUR FUTURE, YOUR LIFE: Taking Responsibility

As a summary to this chapter, we reiterate that a man faced with the possibility of prostate cancer (right from the first DRE that the GP conducts as a part of a routine physical exam), needs to seek out *more than* one opinion on 1) selection of biopsy; 2) selecting the right urologist (if a biopsy is to be performed); 3) understanding the many treatment options (if biopsy results are positive) or, 4) understanding what to do if biopsy results are "negative." (Sometimes, this finding can be as perplexing to the man having night-time symptoms as a positive finding.)

At the risk of over-stating it, the key for any man embarking on this prostate cancer journey is, obviously, to get second and even more, opinions. At the very least, decisions of this magnitude will determine how much longer you may live (with or without cancer), and the quality of your life from this day forward. All those variables and uncertainties require strategic decision-making utilizing the best medical data and doctors' opinions available. It is your responsibility to yourself and to your loved ones. Seek more opinions!

P.S. WHAT ABOUT *YOUR* FAMILY?

We have talked a lot about getting second opinions (and third, forth or more!) and how important it is for the man who's going through the "process" of prostate treatment research and decision-making. What we haven't discussed is, for the man who is married or who has a "significant other" that is part of his life, she will be having just as many fears and questions that need answers and sometimes more! The impact to the "family" of cancer treatment choice can not be understated and a man must deal with those realities up-front.

Fortunately, there are places where information can be obtained to help the whole family deal with prostate cancer. In the ACS book recommended earlier, an entire chapter is devoted to helping find support for the entire family. Among other information, there are support groups for cancer of all types and varieties, but there are support groups for prostate cancer specifically which are listed and detailed in the ACS chapter. However, for our contribution in this Edition 2.0, we will mention only one, called **'US TOO.'**

US TOO was founded in 1990 and is a national organization which is administered by (volunteer) prostate cancer survivors. It has more than 400 chapters with 60,000 members and over 100,000 family members represented throughout the world with headquarters at 930 N. York Road, Suite 50; Hinsdale, IL 60521 and a toll free phone: 800-808-7866. (If those address and phone numbers have changed, check the internet for updated information at **www.ustoo.com/chapters**).

In summary, men need to realize that the impact of prostate problems affects the family, also, and that they are not alone when it comes to seeking help. Through organizations like **US TOO**, families can find they are not alone: help is only a click away on the 'net.

"IF YOU HAVE BEEN DIAGNOSED WITH CANCER (ANY CANCER... NOT *ONLY* PROSTATE CANCER), YOU ABSOLUTELY *MUST* SEEK MORE THAN ONE MEDICAL OPINION ABOUT YOUR TREATMENT OPTIONS! AND, YOU ABSOLUTELY *MUST* SEEK OPINIONS FROM DIFFERENT TREATMENT SPECIALISTS: SURGERY, RADIATION, CRYOGENICS, ROBOTICS SURGERY; ETC."

CHAPTER FOUR

Radical Prostatectomy: Surgical Prostate Removal

Introduction

Radical Prostatectomy has been covered in various other discussions here in this book but it deserves to have its own chapter so that is why this chapter has more details and graphics. It is the most often used treatment for PC but you need to learn about the pros and cons of this 'radical' treatment, in order to be able to make an informed decision about what treatment (if any) is right for you.

Depending upon who you talk to, what doctors and which clinics are visited, the case for surgically removing the prostate is strong. After all, if the cancer is confined to the prostate gland, it seems only logical that cutting it out will cure the cancer, right? So, with this logical thinking in the back of your mind, the question posed to the urologist is: "what would *you* do if this was your diagnosis? What treatment would you do if this was your father or your son, to get the highest probability of success?"

And, usually (but not always), the urologist responds by suggesting that surgery offers the highest and most likely route to success....often times saying something like...*"if you remove the prostate, cancer can usually, never come back..."* (emphasis on "***usually***" intended). And, after all, since urologists specialize in surgery, what kind of response to that question would you expect?

To be fair, there are urologists who urge a patient with that question to pursue other doctor's opinions. Specifically, with the success rate that has been catalogued over the past dozen years or more, from the various radiological treatment procedures that show the 'success' rate is at least equivalent to surgery and, in some studies, slightly better in terms of the 10 year-after-treatment-being-alive criteria for success. So, urologists at this point in time, seem to "get it" and are generally advising their patients to seek out opinions from one or more doctors before making a life-altering decision about which treatment is the best for your particular prostate specific indications.

GOOD NEWS FOR PROSTATECTOMIES

It was mentioned in Chapter Two that robotics have been introduced into the Retropubic Prostatectomy surgery procedures just since about 2000. And, while it is not our intent to endorse a particular clinic or even to recommend a particular procedure for prostate cancer, it is certainly important that we provide you with options and, from our research, names of doctors who have the most experience in any of these procedures.

In the late 1990's the da Vinci laparoscopic (robotic) radical prostatectomy procedure was being pioneered and performed in France. Through the late '90's, clinics in the U.S. and Europe acquired the equipment and began to train surgeons on this precision process for removing the prostate gland. What they learned, through several hundred robot-assisted radical prostatectomies, was that this new robotic technique had a better result when compared with the historical non-robotic surgery procedures then (and now) in more common practice. (You can read about the da Vinci robotics procedure at the end of this Chapter for a more thorough understanding of this state-of-the-art procedure).

Historically, reports in the Journal of Urology (Vol 163, 2000) by Guillonneau and Vallancien and in the same Journal in 2001, Vol 165 peaked interest in the medical community, in the radical prostatectomy/urology robotics technology and clinics from Los Angeles to New York began training and using the method as an alternative to traditional open anatomic RP. One of the first clinics to embrace the da Vinci technique was the Vattikuti Institute at Henry Ford Health Systems in Detroit, Michigan.

Over the years, the Vatti Institute has developed a reputation as a leader in successful robotic-assisted prostatectomies that is rivaled by few other U.S. prostate cancer specialists. Their success, while still too infant to know longevity statistics (i.e. they have been perfoming da Vinci prostatectomies only since 2001), has been reported in papers by the head of their team, Dr. Mani Menon, Ashutosh Tewari, and James Peabody (and their VIP Team members) in the Journal of Urology in both November 2002 and June of 2003. "Success" in the case of the Vatti Institute, is measured in comparison with traditional open anatomic RP's in the following ways:

> ***"Results: In the last 100 cases, mean operative time was 2.5 hours with average blood loss of 150 ml. Median specimen Gleason score was 7 and mean tumor volume was 7 cc....patients were discharged on average, in less than 24 hours and mean catherterization time was 4.2 days. Conclusion: The Vattikuti Institute prostatectomy is a precise and safe minimally invasive technique of radical retropubic prostatectomy..."***
>
> **(M. Menon; et al, Journal of Urology, June 2003).**

When compared with traditional (non-robotic) retropubic RP's, average blood loss is two to three times more than the robot-assisted procedure, hospital duration is 4 to 5 days, catheter duration is measured in weeks, and pain significantly more acute (as reported by retrospective follow-up) for traditional surgery patients. (M. Menon; et al, Journal of Urology, Nov 2002).

But, the biggest problem with the da Vinci procedure is cost. In 2002, the Vitti Institute reported that typical cost of the robot-assisted procedure was approaching $1 Million and insurance companies were not covering it because the data was not yet developed to show it was worth that much. By 2009, the cost had actually fallen to an average of a half million dollars so this shows that we can expect that the fact that more robotics procedures are showing just how much more valuable this procedure is will make it more cost competitive with traditional radical surgery in the next few years.

Part of the reason the costs are so high is, the costs of equipment itself and recurring cost of consumables are almost prohibitive. The procedure takes at least 3 surgeons, not counting the one handling the robotic controls, plus support staff that are highly specialized in the procedure---all of which spells high costs vs. traditional surgery.

Over time, however, those costs will decline and skilled personnel will be trained and available. Consumables and associated operating room costs will decline, also. The time in the hospital will, in some measures, offset follow-up care-costs and the associated support staff and consumables will do the same. Thus, by the time this information is in print, costs may not be such an impediment, although rising health care costs now being borne by the consumer is increasing at the rate of 15% a year, so it remains to be seen.

So, having now set the stage for making the most information available about treatments, this chapter is devoted to providing as much as can be shared about the various radical prostatectomy procedures as can be obtained from clinics and other well respected parishioners in the field, in 2012. Sources of this information (besides the Vatti Institute), include, but are not limited to, the Journal of the American Medical Association (JAMA), the New England Journal of Medicine (NEJM), the National Cancer Institute NCI, the Center for Disease Control (CDC), and numerous journal papers where information on this subject is shared with other peer professionals who are practicing prostate-specific medicine.

Controversy About Long-Term Benefits

A traditional Radical Prostatectomy (retropubic) is performed by making a small incision in the pubic area and surgically removing the prostate. This procedure actually involves peeling away the prostate by layers something that can be described as like peeling an onion, whereby the outer layers of the prostate gland are left attached to the bladder and succhured to surrounding tissue to maintain the bladder structurally for when the prostate has been removed---which formerly was structurally tied to that same surrounding tissue.

The urethra tube that runs from the bladder through the prostate where it picks up seminal fluid that becomes the carrier of the sperm from testicle sack through the penis during sexual ejaculation, must be salvaged and tied to tissue left behind after the prostate is vacated. During this procedure, nerves that were within the prostate and attached to the penis are frequently severed and, unless the surgeon is dedicated to reattaching these, will result in the patient being impotent and/or sexually dysfunctional.

Once the surgery is completed, a catheter will remain in place for a period of 2 to 6 weeks while healing takes place but, nearly 100% of the time, urinary incontinence will follow the removal of the catheter for sometimes as long as a year. For some patients, incontinence is permanent.

Impotence is certain in nearly 100% of radical prostatectomy patients for 6 months to a year following surgery. In many patients, sexual dysfunction is almost a permanent condition although some are able to have sex with use of drugs like Viagra---but, such after effects are very common with the normal surgical process where nerves are sacrificed to remove the prostate gland.

Da Vinci Radical Prostatectomy: A Better Outcome

In the past 10 years, better Radical Prostatectomy procedures have become more common and, along with those, insurance companies have begun to approve them as the costs have come down and nerve-sparing techniques that are much more successful with these minimally-invasive procedures have resulted in a better patient outcome with fewer side-effects that accompany the regular radical surgical procedures.

On the following pages, you will find a description of the De Vinci Radical Prostatectomy procedure, taken from the best sources available who have successfully been treating prostate patients for more than 15 years and reported by the Journal of the American Medical Association and New England Journal of Medicine---two of the best medical Journals in the United States.

JAMA Study: Da Vinci vs Traditional Radical

The following study was performed and written up in the Journal of The American Medical Association in 2009 and clearly shows that the use of the Da Vinci method provides much better long term outcomes for men who chose it over traditional (RPP) surgery. The abstract summary of the paper is included here from JAMA ONLINE:

Comparative Effectiveness of Minimally Invasive vs Open Radical Prostatectomy

Jim C. Hu, MD, MPH; Xiangmei Gu, MS; Stuart R. Lipsitz, ScD; Michael J. Barry, MD; Anthony V. D'Amico, MD, PhD; Aaron C. Weinberg, MD; Nancy L. Keating, MD, MPH

JAMA. 2009;302(14):1557-1564.

ABSTRACT

Context *Minimally* invasive radical prostatectomy (MIRP) has diffused rapidly despite limited data on outcomes and greater costs compared with open retropubic radical prostatectomy (RRP).

Objective To determine the comparative effectiveness of MIRP vs RRP.

Design, Setting, and Patients Population-based observational cohort study using US Surveillance, Epidemiology, and End Results Medicare linked data from 2003 through 2007. We identified men with prostate cancer who underwent MIRP (n = 1938) vs RRP (n = 6899).

Main Outcome Measures We compared postoperative 30-day complications, anastomotic stricture 31 to 365 days postoperatively, long-term incontinence and erectile dysfunction more than 18 months postoperatively, and postoperative use of additional cancer therapies, a surrogate for cancer control.

Results Among men undergoing prostatectomy, use of MIRP increased from 9.2% (95% confidence interval [CI], 8.1%-10.5%) in 2003 to 43.2% (95% CI, 39.6%-46.9%) in 2006-2007. Men undergoing MIRP vs RRP were more likely to be recorded as Asian (6.1% vs 3.2%), less likely to be recorded as black (6.2% vs 7.8%) or Hispanic (5.6% vs 7.9%), and more likely to live in areas with at least 90% high school graduation rates (50.2% vs 41.0%) and with median incomes of at least $60 000 (35.8% vs 21.5%) (all $P < .001$). In propensity score–adjusted analyses, MIRP vs RRP was associated with shorter length of stay (median, 2.0 vs 3.0 days; $P<.001$) and lower rates of blood transfusions (2.7% vs 20.8%; $P < .001$), postoperative respiratory complications (4.3% vs 6.6%; $P = .004$), miscellaneous surgical complications (4.3% vs 5.6%; $P = .03$), and anastomotic stricture (5.8% vs 14.0%; $P < .001$). However, MIRP vs RRP was associated with an increased risk of genitourinary complications (4.7% vs 2.1%; $P = .001$) and diagnoses of incontinence (15.9 vs 12.2 per 100 person-years; $P = .02$) and erectile dysfunction (26.8 vs 19.2 per 100 person-years; $P = .009$). Rates of use of additional cancer therapies did not differ by surgical procedure (8.2 vs 6.9 per 100 person-years; $P = .35$).

Conclusion Men undergoing MIRP vs RRP experienced shorter length of stay, fewer respiratory and miscellaneous surgical complications and strictures, and similar postoperative use of additional cancer therapies but experienced more genitourinary complications, incontinence, and erectile dysfunction.

JAMA Editor' Note: It is clear that fewer side effects involving incontinence and/or sexual impotence accompanies the robotic procedures verses a high incidence of one or both of those side effects occurring when a traditional radical prostatectomy (retropubic) or RRP is conducted. Outcomes appear to be no different: the same life expectancy has been shown for either procedure (i.e. 10 years) but it is not clear how much insurance funding impacts the decision to pursue one or the other surgery type. That was not addressed in this or in any other studies (to date) that compare outcomes of RRP verses Robotics but it can be a factor, particularly where medicare or medicaid are involved.

Objective View of This Study

Many doctors also assume, rightly or not, that a man who is older than (some magic yet unsubstantiated) age is no longer interested in sex so they tend to dismiss this as a reason to choose one type of surgery over another. However, it is clear that a substantial number of men are having sex well into their 70's and should consider the downside of SD when deciding between these two types of radical options----studies are in fact showing that many seniors are enjoying a quality of sex life during their retirement years that hasn't been possible in the previous stress-packed working years before so this is a consideration you need to take into account even if your doctor forgets to ask about it.

Of course, the other downside is urinary incontinence and no man wants to have to wear adult diapers the rest of their lives no matter how that "side effect" is sugar coated when a doctor explains possible after-effects of prostatectemies. This then, needs to be the other discussion point when talking honestly and openly with your doctors about your options. It is also important that you get a second and third opinion from other doctors who perform either or both of these types of radical surgeries---you may be surprised at differences in the various doctor's willingness to give you details and it can only help you make a good decision for the treatment that is right for you.

da Vinci Method Explained

With *da Vinci,* small incisions are used to introduce miniaturized wristed instruments and a high-definition 3D camera. Seated comfortably at the *da Vinci* console, the surgeon views a magnified, high-resolution 3D image of the surgical site.

At the same time, state-of-the-art robotic and computer technologies scale, filter and seamlessly translate your surgeon's hand movements into precise micro-movements of the *da Vinci* instruments.

The System cannot be programmed, nor can it make decisions on its own. Rather, the *da Vinci* System requires that every surgical maneuver be performed with direct input from your surgeon.

da Vinci Surgical System consists of an ergonomically designed surgeon's console, a patient cart with four interactive robotic arms, a high-performance vision System and patented *EndoWrist* instruments.

(From the da Vinci SurgiSystem website):

At the *da Vinci* console, your surgeon operates while seated comfortably, viewing a highly magnified 3D image of the body's interior. To operate, the surgeon uses master controls that work like forceps.

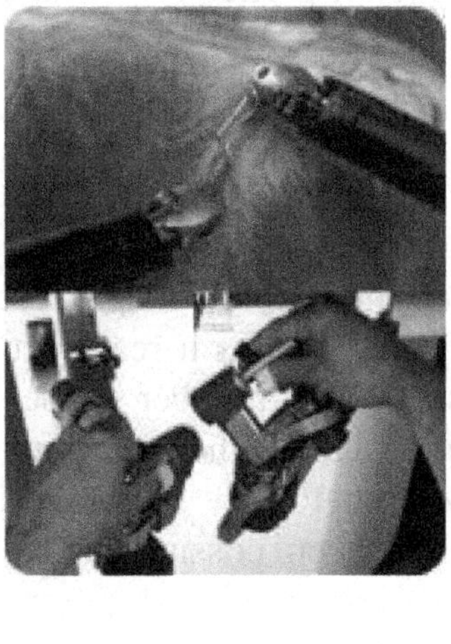

As your surgeon manipulates the controls, *da Vinci* responds to your surgeon's input in real time, translating his or her hand, wrist and finger movements into precise movements of miniaturized instruments at the patient-side cart.

At the *da Vinci* console, the surgeon operates while seated comfortably, viewing a highly magnified 3D image of the body's interior. To operate, the surgeon uses master controls that work like forceps.

As the surgeon manipulates the controls, *da Vinci* responds to the surgeon's input in real time, translating his or her hand, wrist and finger movements into precise movements of miniaturized instruments at the patient-side cart.

The *da Vinci*'s patient cart holds up to three *EndoWrist* instruments and one 3D camera. To access the target anatomy, the surgeon introduces the precisly controlled *EndoWrist* instruments into the body through a series of dime-sized incisions. A broad range of instrument types are available to help the surgeon perform specialized surgical tasks with precision and control.

Urologic Surgery

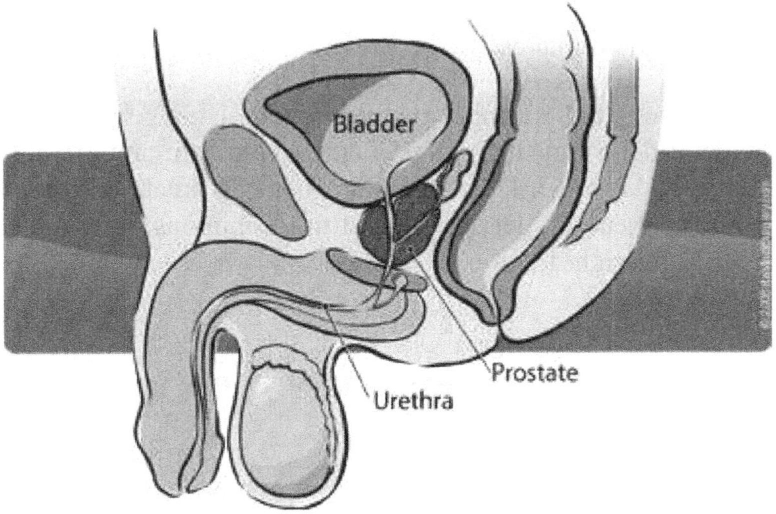

When medication and other non-surgical treatments are unavailable or cannot relieve symptoms, surgery is the recommended treatment for many conditions that affect the male reproductive organs and urinary tract organs. These conditions include, among other things, prostate cancer, ureteropelvic junction (UPJ) obstruction, bladder and kidney cancer and vesicoureteral reflux.

Facing urologic surgery can create a great deal of anxiety. Typically, a common concern is: "Will my body function normally after surgery?" Traditional open urologic surgery using large incisions to access the pelvic organs has been the standard approach when surgery is needed. But there are several drawbacks to this procedure including: significant post-surgical pain, a long recovery and an unpredictable and potentially long-term impact on continence and sexual function.

Fortunately, less invasive surgical options are available to many people facing urologic surgery. The most common is laparoscopy, which uses small incisions. Laparoscopy can be very effective for many routine procedures, but limitations of this technology prevent its use for more complex urologic surgeries.

A new category of surgery, the *da Vinci* ® Surgical System, is being used by an increasing number of surgeons worldwide for prostatectomy and other urologic procedures. It is a minimally invasive approach, using the latest in surgical and robotics technologies and is ideal for delicate urologic surgery. This includes prostatectomy, where the target site is not only tightly confined but also surrounded by nerves affecting urinary control and sexual function.

Using *da Vinci* , a surgeon has a better tool to spare those delicate and critical surrounding nerves. This may or may not improve the recovery experience and clinical outcomes with such benefits as:

- Significantly less pain
- Less blood loss
- Fewer complications
- Less scarring
- A shorter hospital stay
- And a faster return to normal daily activities

As with any surgery, these benefits cannot be guaranteed, as surgery is unique to each patient and procedure. The da Vinci Surgical System is considered safe and effective, but may not be appropriate for everyone. Always ask your doctor about all treatment options, as well as the benefits and risks. And, remember, get second and third opinions before deciding if surgery or other treatment regime is the right for you.

Treatment Comparison

- Surgery vs. Radiotherapy
- da Vinci ® vs. Open Surgery & Laparoscopy
- Key Comparative Studies

Surgery vs. Radiotherapy

The following table compares outcomes following prostate cancer treatment — specifically, surgery (radical prostatectomy), which is considered the gold standard treatment for localized prostate cancer — and radiation (external beam radiation). Data is provided on survival, cancer recurrence, incidence of rectal and bladder cancer, bowel function, urinary issues and long-term erectile function.

In this table, radical prostatectomy includes all approaches to prostate surgery (open surgery through large incisions; conventional minimally invasive, or laparoscopic radical prostatectomy – also called LRP – as well as da Vinci Prostatectomy, or dVP). As you can see, surgery offers measurable advantages over external beam radiation in terms of outcomes and survivability. No comparison is made here for brachytherapy outcomes.

Outcome Comparison: Surgery vs. Radiotherapy		
Outcome	**Radical Prostatectomy***	**Radiation****
Survival duration compared to conservative disease management[1]	8.6 years	4.6 years
15-year prostate cancer survival rate[2]	92%	87%
Survival rate for high-grade cancer patients[3]	45% increase in overall survival rate vs. radiotherapy	-
Risk of cancer-specific death for high-grade cancer patients[4]	49% less risk vs. radiotherapy	-
Cancer recurrence[5]	Easy to detect	Difficult to detect
Risk of rectal cancer (Within 10 year follow-up)[6]	5.1 out of 1000	10 out of 1000
Risk of bladder cancer[7]	0.8% develop bladder cancer	1.3% developed bladder cancer
Bowel function impairment[8]	-	Significantly greater vs. surgery
Disease-specific long-term quality of life[9]	Stable	Unstable
Painful urination (at 18 month follow-up)[10]	1% of patients	30% of patients
Long-term erectile dysfunction[11]	Lower risk	Higher risk

*Open surgery; comparable long-term data not yet available on da Vinci Prostatectomy.

**External Beam Radiation Therapy (EBRT) unless otherwise noted in the citation.

da Vinci vs. Open Surgery & Laparoscopy

The following table looks at patient outcomes following surgery for prostate cancer (radical prostatectomy), and compares "best in class" data from three types of surgery. As you can see, da Vinci Prostatectomy (dVP) shows measurable advantages as compared to both conventional open surgery (open), performed through large incisions, as well as conventional minimally invasive laparoscopic (lap) surgery.

da Vinci® vs. Open vs. Conventional Laparoscopy			
Outcome	*da Vinci®*	Open	Lap
Cancer control			
T2 margin status	2.5[1]	5.9[2]	7.7[3]
Complications			
Estimated blood loss (EBL)	109 ml[4]	1355 ml[5]	380 ml[6]
Length of stay (LOS)	1.2 days[4]	3 days[5]	2.5 days[13]
Major	1.7%[4]	6.7%[5]	3.7[6]
Minor	3.7%[4]	12.6%[5]	14.6%[6]
Urinary function			
3 month	92.9%[7]	54%[8]	62%[9]
6 month	94.9%[7]	80%[8]	77%[9]
12 month	97.4%[7]	93%[8]	83%[9]
Sexual function			
12 month	86%[10]	71%[11]	76%[12]

*Two Key Comparative Studies Support Robotic Prostatectomies

1. Long-term survival probability in men with clinically localized prostate cancer treated either conservatively or with definitive treatment (radiotherapy or radical prostatectomy)

Ashutosh Tewaria, Jay D. Ramana, Peter Changa, Sandhya Raoa, George Divineb and Mani Menon
Urology, Volume 68, Issue 6, December 2006, Pages 1268-1274

Objectives:

To report the long-term survival probability in more than 3000 men with localized prostate cancer treated either conservatively or by definitive treatment (radiotherapy or radical prostatectomy).

Methods:

We studied 3159 men with biopsy-confirmed, clinically localized prostate cancer diagnosed from 1980 to 1997. We restricted our analysis to men 75 years of age or younger. The extent of comorbid disease was measured using the Charlson score. The Cox proportional hazards regression model was used to compare long-term survival in patients who were treated conservatively versus survival in patients treated with either radiotherapy or radical prostatectomy.

Results:

After adjusting for age, race, tumor grade, comorbid disease, income status, and year of diagnosis, the overall survival rate at 15 years was 35% for conservative management, 50% for radiotherapy, and 65% for radical prostatectomy. The corresponding prostate cancer-specific survival rates were 79%, 87%, and 92%. Patients undergoing radiotherapy or radical prostatectomy had lower overall mortality than patients undergoing conservative management (adjusted relative risk 0.67 for radiotherapy and 0.41 for prostatectomy; $P < 0.001$). The increase in the survival duration was 4.6 years with radiotherapy and 8.6 years with radical prostatectomy.

Conclusions:

The authors note that the results of this study have shown that compared with conservative management, both radiotherapy and radical prostatectomy increase survival for men with localized prostate cancer.

2. Long-Term Survival in Men With High Grade Prostate Cancer: A Comparison Between Conservative Treatment, Radiation Therapy and Radical Prostatectomy—A Propensity Scoring Approach

Ashutosh Tewarin, George Divine, Peter Chang, M. Mendel Shemtov, Matthew Milowsky, David Nanus and Mani Menon
The Journal of Urology, Volume 177, Issue 3, March 2007, Pages 911-915

Purpose:

We performed a retrospective cohort study using propensity score analysis to calculate long-term survival in patients with prostate cancer with Gleason score 8 or greater who were treated with conservative therapy, radiation therapy and radical prostatectomy.

Materials and Methods:

Between January 1, 1980 and December 31, 1997, 3,159 patients in the Henry Ford Health System were diagnosed with clinically localized prostate cancer (i.e. cancer contained within the prostate gland). Of these patients 453 had a Gleason score of 8 or greater in the biopsy specimen and they were the cohort. The end points were overall and prostate cancer specific survival. Propensity score analysis was used to more precisely compare the 3 treatments of observation, radiation and radical prostatectomy. Median patient followup was longer in the radical prostatectomy arm than in the conservative treatment and radiation therapy arms (68 months vs 52 and 54, respectively).

Results:

Of the 453 patients 197 (44%) were treated conservatively, 137 (30%) received radiation therapy and 119 (26%) underwent radical prostatectomy. Using propensity scoring analysis median overall survival for conservative therapy, radiation and radical prostatectomy was 5.2, 6.7 and 9.7 years, respectively. Median cancer specific survival was 7.8 years for conservative therapy and more than 14 years for radiation therapy and radical prostatectomy. The risk of cancer specific death following radical prostatectomy was 68% lower than for conservative treatment and 49% lower than for radiation therapy ($p < 0.001$ and 0.053, respectively).

Conclusions:

Survival of men with high grade prostate cancer can be improved by radical prostatectomy or radiation therapy.

Conclusions here are from the two studies quoted, plus information taken directly from the da Vinci website where the da Vinci Method explanation is drawn from. The information provided here is neither endorsed or supported by the author(s) of* ***Prostate Cancer 2.0**; it is provided here for information only.*

Other References From These Studies You May Want To Review:

1. Tewari A, Raman JD, Chang P, Rao S, Divine G, Menon M. Long-term survival probability in men with clinically localized prostate cancer treated either conservatively or with definitive treatment (radiotherapy or radical prostatectomy). Urology. 2006 Dec;68(6):1268-74.
2. Tewari A, Raman JD, Chang P, Rao S, Divine G, Menon M. Long-term survival probability in men with clinically localized prostate cancer treated either conservatively or with definitive treatment (radiotherapy or radical prostatectomy). Urology. 2006 Dec;68(6):1268-74.
3. Tewari A, Divine G, Chang P, Shemtov MM, Milowsky M, Nanus D, Menon M. Long-term survival in men with high grade prostate cancer: a comparison between conservative treatment, radiation therapy and radical prostatectomy--a propensity scoring approach. J Urol. 2007 Mar;177(3):911-5. Erratum in: J Urol. 2007 May;177(5):1958.
4. Tewari A, Divine G, Chang P, Shemtov MM, Milowsky M, Nanus D, Menon M. Long-term survival in men with high grade prostate cancer: a comparison between conservative treatment, radiation therapy and radical prostatectomy--a propensity scoring approach. J Urol. 2007 Mar;177(3):911-5. Erratum in: J Urol. 2007 May;177(5):1958.
5. Di Blasio, C. J., A. C. Rhee, et al. (2003). Predicting clinical end points: treatment nomograms in prostate cancer. Semin Oncol 30(5): 567-86.
6. Baxter NN, Tepper JE, Durham SB, Rothenberger DA, Virnig BA. Increased risk of rectal cancer after prostate radiation: a population-based study. Gastroenterology. 2005 Apr;128(4):819-24.
7. Boorjian S, Cowan JE, Konety BR, DuChane J, Tewari A, Carroll PR, Kane CJ; Cancer of the Prostate Strategic Urologic Research Endeavor Investigators. Bladder cancer incidence and risk factors in men with prostate cancer: results from Cancer of the Prostate Strategic Urologic Research Endeavor. J Urol. 2007 Mar;177(3):883-7; discussion 887-8.
8. Litwin MS, Sadetsky N, Pasta DJ, Lubeck DP. Bowel function and bother after treatment for early stage prostate cancer: a longitudinal quality of life analysis from CaPSURE. J Urol. 2004 Aug;172(2):515-9.
9. Miller, D. C., M. G. Sanda, et al. (2005). Long-term outcomes among localized prostate cancer survivors: health-related quality-of-life changes after radical prostatectomy, external radiation, and brachytherapy. J Clin Oncol 23(12): 2772-80.

10. Buron, C., B. Le Vu, et al. (2007). Brachytherapy versus prostatectomy in localized prostate cancer: Results of a French multicenter prospective medico-economic study. Int J Radiat Oncol Biol Phys 67(3): 812-22.
11. Di Blasio, C. J., A. C. Rhee, et al. (2003). Predicting clinical end points: treatment nomograms in prostate cancer. Semin Oncol 30(5): 567-86.

References for Chart 2:

1. Patel VR, Thaly R, Shah K.Robotic radical prostatectomy: outcomes of 500 cases. BJU Int. 2007 May;99(5):1109-12.
2. Scardino PT. Open Radical Retropubic Prostatectomy. Presented at the American Urological Association's Carcinoma of the Prostate Course , San Francisco, California, Sept. 30 – Oct. 1 2005
3. Touijer K, Kuroiwa K, Saranchuk JW, Hassen WA, Trabulsi EJ, Reuter VE, Guillonneau B. Quality improvement in laparoscopic radical prostatectomy for pT2 prostate cancer: impact of video documentation review on positive surgical margin. J Urol. 2005 Mar;173(3):765-8. p. 766 (Results)
4. Bhandari, A., McIntire, L., Kaul, S.A., Hemal, A.K., Peabody, J.O., and Menon, M. (2005). Perioperative complications of robotic radical prostatectomy after the learning curve. J Urol 174, 915-918.
5. Brown, J.A., Garlitz, C., Gomella, L.G., McGinnis, D.E., Diamond, S.M., and Strup, S.E. (2004). Perioperative morbidity of laparoscopic radical prostatectomy compared with open radical retropubic prostatectomy. Urologic oncology 22, 102-106.
6. Guillonneau, B., Rozet, F., Cathelineau, X., Lay, F., Barret, E., Doublet, J.D., Baumert, H., and Vallancien, G. (2002). Perioperative complications of laparoscopic radical prostatectomy: the Montsouris 3-year experience. The Journal of urology 167, 51-56.
7. Locke, DR, Klimberg IW and Sessions RP. Robotic Radical Prostatectomy With Continence And Potency Sparing Technique: An Analysis Of The First 250 Cases. Submitted To Journal Of Urology, Publication Date TBD. p. 5 table 4.
8. Walsh PC. Patient-reported urinary continence and sexual function after anatomic radical prostatectomy. J Urol. 2000 Jul;164(1):242. p. 59 table 1.
9. Goeman, L., Salomon, L., La De Taille, A., Vordos, D., Hoznek, A., Yiou, R., and Abbou, C.C. (2006). Long-term functional and oncological results after retroperitoneal laparoscopic prostatectomy according to a prospective evaluation of 550 patients. World J Urol 24, 281-288.
10. Kaul, S., Bhandari, A., Hemal, A., Savera, A., Shrivastava, A., and Menon, M. (2005). Robotic radical prostatectomy with preservation of the prostatic fascia: a feasibility study. Urology 66, 1261-1265.
11. Parsons JK, Marschke P, Maples P, Walsh PC. Effect of methylprednisolone on return of sexual function after nerve-sparing radical retropubic prostatectomy. Urology. 2004 Nov;64(5):987-90.
12. Su, L.M., Link, R.E., Bhayani, S.B., Sullivan, W., and Pavlovich, C.P. (2004). Nerve-sparing laparoscopic radical prostatectomy: replicating the open surgical technique. Urology 64, 123
13. Dahl DM, L'esperance JO, Trainer AF, Jiang Z, Gallagher K, Litwin DE, Blute RD Jr. "Laparoscopic radical prostatectomy: initial 70 cases at a U.S. university medical center."Urology. 2002 Nov;60(5):859-63.

From the da Vinci Website: Disclaimer:

While clinical studies support the effectiveness of the *da Vinci*® System when used in minimally invasive surgery, individual results may vary. Surgery with the *da Vinci* Surgical System may not be appropriate for every individual. Always ask your doctor about all treatment options, as well as their risks and benefits.

Other Views and Other Studies about Robotic Prostatectomies:

'...Review: New prostate surgery not necessarily better'---

JAMA Study: Incontinence and ED More Likely But Hospital stays shorter with less-invasive surgery*

*** Incontinence, impotence more common with newer approach***

By Julie Steenhuysen

CHICAGO, Oct 13, 2009 (Reuters) - Men who have less invasive prostate cancer surgery -- often done robotically -- are more likely to be incontinent and have erectile dysfunction (ED) than men who have conventional open surgery, U.S. researchers said on Tuesday.

Many men, especially those who are wealthy and highly educated, favor minimally invasive surgery because they assume the high-tech approach will yield better results, but the evidence on that is mixed, the team reported in the Journal of the American Medical Association.

"We found men undergoing minimally invasive versus open surgery were more likely to have a diagnosis of incontinence and erectile dysfunction," Dr. Jim Hu of Brigham and Women's Hospital in Boston said in a telephone briefing.

Hu said use of minimally invasive surgery has taken off since the introduction and heavy marketing of robot-assisted surgery, such as the da Vinci system made by Intuitive Surgical Inc (ISRG.O).

The system consists of robotic arms, controlled from a console, that allow surgeons to perform less invasive surgeries. Hospitals advertise the systems as being able to reduce trauma, blood loss, risk of infection, scarring and often pain.

Hu said so far, there have been few studies that compare minimally invasive surgery with open surgery.

To do that, he and colleagues used billing data from the Medicare insurance program for the elderly on procedures done from 2003 to 2007. During that time, use of minimally invasive surgery for prostate cancer increased fivefold.

While both approaches fared equally well as a cancer treatment, they found that men who got the minimally invasive approach had shorter hospital stays, were less likely to need blood transfusions, and had fewer breathing problems after surgery than those who got conventional surgery.

But they were also more likely to have complications involving the genital and urinary organs, and they were more often diagnosed as having incontinence and erectile dysfunction than men who got open surgery.

The researchers also noted that fewer black and Hispanic men had the minimally invasive surgery, while Asians were much more likely to get the high-tech surgery.

CHOICE RELATED TO EDUCATION, WEALTH

Men who got the minimally invasive surgery were far more likely to live in areas with at least 90 percent high school graduation rates and median income of at least $60,000.

The fact that highly educated, wealthier men favored the higher technology alternative "despite insufficient data demonstrating superiority" may reflect a healthcare system "enamored with new technology" that increases health costs without offering clear benefits, Hu and colleagues wrote.

Ryan Rhodes, marketing director for Intuitive Surgical, disputed the findings.

"There have been over 800 papers (as of October 2009) published in peer reviewed journals talking about the outcomes of radical prostatectomy. The majority of these were favorable," Rhodes said.

He said the JAMA study used Medicare billing data, which does not distinguish between robot-assisted and other types of minimally invasive prostate surgery.

"Looking at the data, you cannot accurately assess which patients were operated on robotically," he said.

Dr. Herbert Lepor of New York University's Langone Medical Center analyzed several studies on robotic-assisted prostate surgery in a paper published this year in Reviews in Urology. He said so far the evidence does not suggest the robotic procedure is superior to open surgery.

Lepor, who was not involved in the study, estimates that about 80 percent of minimally invasive prostate cancer surgery is done robotically. "What drives this is the industry creating the need," he said.

"We've increased the cost of care with the robot," he said. "Now what we are learning is continence and potency seem to be inferior."

(Editing by Maggie Fox and Mohammad Zargham for Reuters Health)

OTHER SOURCES OF INFORMATION ABOUT ROBOTICS

In addition to Journal information, it is important to know what others are saying about Prostate Cancer treatment today. Here are a few of the articles in the popular press that will give you a better picture of how effective robotics-assisted PC surgery is:

Is robot prostate surgery best for quality of life?

By Amy Norton

Apr 5, 2010

NEW YORK (Reuters Health) - Despite the popularity of robot-assisted procedures for prostate cancer, when it comes to men's long-term quality of life, patients with earlier stage cancers generally fare better with non-surgical approaches than with surgery, according to a new study.

Researchers say the findings, reported in the **May, 2010** ***Journal of Urology***, offer men more information to consider when deciding on treatment.

Men with earlier stage prostate cancer have a number of treatment options, from "watchful waiting" to radiation to surgical removal of the prostate gland.

When it comes to surgery, robot-assisted laparoscopic surgery -- where the surgeon sits at a console, operating robotic "arms" that extract the prostate gland through small cuts in the abdomen -- has become the dominant approach in the U.S.

After hospitals invest the roughly $1.5 million for the machines, plus the costs of surgeon training and annual service contracts, they often aggressively market robotic surgery. That may include claims that it carries lower risks of long-term incontinence and impotence than traditional open surgery. Actual study data to prove that, however, are lacking.

In the new study, researchers at the Sentara Health System/Eastern Virginia Medical School in Norfolk followed 785 men who received one of four types of treatment for localized prostate cancer (cancer confined to prostate gland) at their center between 2000 and 2008.

Overall, 135 men underwent traditional "open" surgery to remove the prostate gland, while 447 had robotic surgery. Another 122 patients had brachytherapy, or radioactive "seeds" implanted in the prostate gland to kill the cancer cells. The remaining 81 patients had cryotherapy, where the doctor uses thin metal rods inserted through the perineum to freeze prostate gland tissue and kill the resident cancer cells.

In general, the researchers found, men treated with radioactive seeds tended to fare best in terms of quality of life, based on standardized questionnaires they completed before treatment and periodically for three years afterward.

Patients who had received either radioactive seeds or cryotherapy had higher average scores when it came to urinary function, versus men who had either type of surgery. And together, men who had radioactive seed implants or cryotherapy were three times as likely as surgery patients to return to at least 90 percent of their pre-treatment score for urinary function.

When it came to sexual function, radioactive seed patients reported a greater quality of life than those who had received any of the other three treatments. Three years after treatment, radioactive seed patients' scores for sexual function and "bother" -- the degree to which they thought their sexual side effects were a problem -- were higher than they were before treatment.

In contrast, scores remained below pre-treatment levels for men in each of the other treatment groups. Cryotherapy patients had the poorest scores long term.

However, there were no significant differences in quality of life between men who had undergone open surgery and those who'd had robot-assisted surgery.

"I think data like these give men more information to use in their decision-making," Dr. Michael D. Fabrizio, one of the researchers on the study, said in an interview.

As for the lack of difference between open and robotic surgery, Fabrizio said that while there are advantages to the robot -- including far less blood loss during surgery and shorter hospital stays -- that may not necessarily translate into better long-term quality of life.

He noted that there is a "big push" to promote robotic surgery, and many patients "assume it's the way to go."

But the current findings, the researchers write in their report, "serve as a reminder that popular enthusiasm for robotic prostatectomy merits temperance."

Nor do the findings come down in favor of any single therapy, however. "This study doesn't tell patients what's right for everyone," said lead researcher Dr. John B. Malcolm, and men still have to talk with their doctors about which treatment might be best for them.

The study did not look at the four treatments' effectiveness against the cancer, Malcolm told Reuters Health, but other research has suggested that surgery is more effective than radioactive seeds.

The study had a number of limitations as well, including a lack of information on any other patient health problems that might have been affecting their sexual or urinary function.

It was also not designed as a randomized, controlled clinical trial -- where patients are randomly assigned to receive a particular treatment, notes Dr. Stephan A. Boorjian, of Fox Chase Cancer Center in Philadelphia, in a commentary published with the study. Such trials are considered the gold standard for assessing a given treatment's outcomes.

A second commentary says that the findings point to a broader issue: the general lack of randomized clinical trials comparing prostate cancer treatments with each other -- in terms of cancer control or quality of life.

"If the standard for evaluating all treatments for prostate cancer were raised," writes Dr. Yair Lotan, of the University of Texas Southwestern Medical Center in Dallas, "then patients and physicians would be able to use more objective criteria in determining the optimal treatment."

SOURCE: Journal of Urology, published ONLINE, May 2010.

More robotics articles....

Is newer prostate surgery really better than the old?

By Rachael Myers Lowe
Feb 22, 2010

NEW YORK (Reuters Health) - Robot-assisted laparoscopic, or "keyhole," surgery appears to be no better at reducing side effects than traditional "open" surgery to remove a cancerous prostate gland, according to new study from Memorial Sloan-Kettering Cancer Center in New York. Critics, however, claim the study relied on old data that doesn't reflect current practice. (February, 2010)

Typically, in traditional open radical prostatectomy, a 6-inch long incision is made in the abdomen and the walnut-sized prostate gland and nearby lymph nodes are removed.

With the newer laparoscopic radical prostatectomy (LRP), several small incisions are made in the lower abdomen through which long-armed surgical instruments, including a camera, are inserted. While watching on a monitor, the surgeon manipulates the tools to cut away and extract the cancerous prostate and other tissue. Most laparoscopic surgeries performed today are robot-assisted.

While robot-assisted LRP usually leads to less blood loss and time spent in the hospital, the high cost of the equipment, its annual maintenance, and a long learning curve for surgeons has raised questions about its value, especially if patient outcomes are no better than the gold standard open surgery.

To investigate, Dr. William T. Lowrance and colleagues analyzed the outcomes for 5,923 men who had surgery to remove the prostate between 2003 and 2005. Overall, 4,858 men (82 percent) had the open procedure and 1,065 (18 percent) had the less-invasive LRP procedure. The claims data did not distinguish between LRP and robot-assisted LRP.

According to a report in The Journal of Urology, there were no differences between the older open procedure and the newer laparoscopic procedure in terms of deaths or medical or surgical complications 90 days after surgery, nor in use of additional cancer therapies in the year after surgery.

Yet, the researchers report that hospital advertising of LRP services was widespread and often overstated and implied benefits "not currently supported by existing evidence."

"It's perfectly reasonable for a man today to want a robot-assisted laparoscopic prostatectomy but patients need to have realistic expectations," which may be lacking, Lowrance told Reuters Health in an interview.

In a commentary published with the study, Dr. Yair Lotan, a cancer surgeon at the University of Texas Southwestern Medical Center in Dallas, wrote that the level of experience of the surgeon performing the procedure is more important for patient outcome than the type of procedure itself.

Lotan thinks patients "should be educated on likely outcomes of a procedure based on individual surgeon experience."

Dr. Jason Engel, Director of Urologic Robotic Surgery at George Washington University Hospital in Washington, D.C., agrees that surgeon experience is key to patient outcomes. He performs about 200 robot-assisted LRPs every year.

The Lowrance study, Engel told Reuters Health, is based on old data that does not reflect the level of surgeon expertise in robot-assisted LRP that is common today. In addition, the Medicare claims used in the study did not distinguish between patients who got the older LRP procedure and the new robot-assisted method.

"Nobody does the old LRP procedure any more," he said. "It's like comparing apples and oranges."

He acknowledged that some institutions over-sell the benefits of the robot-assisted LRP but he defended honest marketing campaigns.

"If I'm doing a great job, how am I going to get my name out there to let people realize there is this great product, when everyone knows to just go to an established institution, like Johns Hopkins, which specializes in the open RP (radical prostatectomy)," Engel said.

Engel also predicted that looking at data from surgeries performed more recently will likely show a difference in outcomes favoring robot-assisted LRP. The Lowrance study hinted at it, he noted, by finding no difference in outcomes at a time when surgeons were just starting to build experience.

"There's never been a head-to-head comparison between an experienced open surgeon and experienced robotic surgeon," Engel told Reuters Health.

Lotan believes the exponential growth of robot-assisted LRP services has been driven by a particularly American phenomenon - the perception that the newest high-tech procedures are the best even if supporting evidence is lacking.

Hospitals, noted Lotan, rarely recoup the millions of dollars spent on the robot equipment and its upkeep, but must have it to attract doctors and patients to their institutions.

Prostate cancer is the most commonly diagnosed cancer in American men. According to the American Cancer Society, more than 192,000 Americans are diagnosed with the disease annually; more than half are over the age 65.

SOURCE: The Journal of Urology, published online February 22, 2010.

...And, a more comprehensive paper about Robotics Prostatectomies...

Nerve Sparing Robotic Prostatectomy: A Novel and Minimally Invasive Treatment of Prostate Cancer

(PCRI Insights: November 2004, vol. 7, no. 4)

By **Ashutosh Tewari, MD**, Director Robotic Oncology and Prostate Cancer Outcomes at Weill Cornell Medical School, New York Presbyterian Hospital, and **Mani Menon, MD**, Director of Vattikuti Institute of Urology, Henry Ford Hospital, Detroit, MI

Supported by: Akshay Bhandari, MD, Sanjeev Kaul, MD, James Peabody, MD, Alok Shrivastava, MD, Ashok Hemal, MD, Melissa Fisher, MD and Kurshid Guru, MD

Introduction

Recent developments in the field of surgical robotics have ushered in a new era of minimally invasive surgery that now challenges conventional open surgery.

Currently available telemanipulation devices allow the performance of complex surgical tasks with dexterity and minimal fatigue due to their ergonomic design, expanded degree of movements, tremor filtering, and 3-D stereoscopic visualization. These devices provide an unsurpassable view of the operative field and unrestricted ability to execute any surgical task. Robotic surgery has been embraced by urologists who have applied it to complex surgical procedures such as pyeloplasty, radical cystectomy, donor nephrectomy, and radical prostatectomy.[2-4]

Background

Goals of treatment: The goal of treating prostate cancer includes complete eradication of cancer coupled with minimal morbidity and negligible deterioration of quality of life. In order to meet these goals, we use a da Vinci master-slave robot system and have developed a minimally invasive, robot-assisted radical prostatectomy technique. This is accomplished (1) by standardizing a unique sequence of surgical steps, appropriate visual angles using different lenses, optimal retraction strategies, precise suturing steps, and anatomical sparing of the neurovascular structures and (2) by incorporating time-tested open surgical principles.[5,6] This technique (which we call the VIP technique) results in excellent oncological and surgical outcomes; causes minimal bleeding, and can be completed in 90 to 160 minutes. The patient satisfaction has been tremendous. Not only do both patients and families appreciate the cosmetic benefits, but also hospitalization has been significantly reduced. Most patients can revert back to their normal lifestyle in less than two weeks.

Dr. Menon developed the technique in Detroit at the Vattikuti Institute of Urology and it has been popularized at several centers in the USA. The data presented here is based on published data from Henry Ford Hospital.[5,7-16]

Patient selection:. Men with clinically localized prostate cancer who choose surgical treatment are candidates for this procedure. The authors use survival prediction tables for selecting patients for surgical treatment. The data has been published[17] by the authors and is available online at: www.prostatecalculator.org/survival.html.

Patients undergo a thorough preoperative evaluation including serum PSA testing, an international prostate symptom score (IPSS), a sexual function inventory, a quality of life score, and an incontinence questionnaire. We also record information about other co-morbidities, such as stroke, cerebral aneurysm, diabetes mellitus, hypertension, COPD (chronic obstructive pulmonary disease) and history of myocardial infarctions.

We specifically question each patient regarding his medical history, with emphasis on abdominal surgery, peritonitis, knee or hip surgery, or peripheral neuropathy. Previous abdominal surgery is not a contraindication. However, a history of stroke or cerebral aneurysm is a relative contraindication for this procedure, since, for 1-3 hours, the patient would be placed in a pronounced Trendelenberg position, in which he is placed head down on a table inclined at about 45° from the floor with the knees uppermost and the legs hanging over the end of the table.

Patients are admitted on the day of surgery and receive deep vein thrombosis (DVT) prophylaxis (Heparin 5000 IU SC on call to the operating room) and an antibiotic in the preoperative holding. Venodyne boots, which gently compress the patient's legs during surgery to prevent postoperative embolic problems, are placed and the abdomen is shaved from nipple to groin.

Procedure: The opening in the bladder is sutured to the end of the urethra to re- create the continuity. The endo wrist technology and magnified 3-D vision maximizes precision and allows anastomosis (suturing) to be more secure and watertight.

We try to avoid damaging the muscles surrounding the urethra and thus leave the sphincter intact. This enables early return of urinary control. We also preserve maximum blood supply to the urethra and other surrounding structures by precisely suturing only those vessels that are entering the prostate and are absolutely required for the safe removal of the cancerous gland. We attempt to identify any local spread by use of frozen sections and take counter measures to maximize cancer control.

Retrieval of specimen and completion of surgery: The cancer containing prostate gland is entrapped (intact) in a thick plastic bag to avoid any tumor spillage. We remove the specimen after slightly enlarging the umbilical incision as required, and we use plastic steri-strips for surgical closure of the incisions.

Postoperative care and discharge: The patients are sent to recovery on intravenous fluids, antibiotics and pain meds. They usually are walking on the evening of the operation and go home either on the same day or the next morning. The catheter is removed between 4-7 days after surgery. It is rare to use blood transfusions in this procedure, and the post-operative pain is minimal. Patients have small cosmetic incisions, and they go back to their work in approximately 12-14 days. Many patients, who are from distant places fly back to their homes in 1-2 days.

Contemporary Results: From a patient perspective,[19] the following concerns have been reported to have the most influence on prostate cancer therapy: oncological control (margin and PSA recurrence), pain, complications, convenience (catheter duration and hospital stay) and functional outcomes (incontinence and sexual recovery). Herein, we analyze the results of our published series of patients treated with robotic prostatectomy in comparison with open radical retropubic prostatectomy (RRP),[13] bearing in mind the aforementioned patients' key preference points. The following discussion is based on this work.[4] Table 1 shows that the baseline patients' characteristics in both groups were comparable.

Continence: Based on third party telephone interviews, we used survival analysis to compute the probability of return of continence by two groups of the patients. Robotic prostatectomy patients achieved continence much more quickly than RRP patients; achieving a 50% return of continence required 160 days in RRP arm as opposed to 44 days in robotic prostatectomy patients ($p<0.05$).[11]

Sexual Function: The sexual function was also evaluated using third party telephone interviews. The response was compiled as the ability to (1) achieve erections and (2) maintain erections adequate for intercourse. The analysis was limited to (1) patients who classified themselves as having normal preoperative erections and sexual intercourse and (2) the ones who underwent bilateral nerve sparing. The response indicated that robotic prostatectomy patients' erections returned more than twice as quickly [50% return of erection occurred at mean follow-up of 180 days vs. 440 days for RRP patients ($p<0.05$)]. The return of intercourse was also quicker in the robotic prostatectomy group in which 50% patients achieved intercourse at a mean follow-up of 340 days. Conversely, the RRP patients have not yet achieved 50% return of intercourse at 700 days ($p<0.05$). Forty two percent of robotic prostatectomy and 65% of RRP patients were known to be using Sildenafil (Viagra®) at the time of analysis.[11]

Operative Comparisons: The robotic prostatectomy patients needed an extra 15 minutes for the setup, but the overall operative times were comparable in two groups. On the other hand, the blood loss of the robotic prostatectomy patients was one-tenth that of the RRP patients. Using this technique, a trained robotic team can perform 3-6 cases a day.

Robotic versus Laparoscopic Prostatectomy

In laparoscopy, the surgeon uses long instruments through small openings and maneuvers them with direct hand contact. Robotic systems use even more delicate instruments that possess two additional degrees of movement excursion (for a total of six, as with a human hand). Comfortably seated at the robot console, the surgeon can maneuver the instruments via a computer interface.

Laparoscopic radical prostatectomy is associated with a steep learning curve. Even in the hands of expert surgeons, laparoscopic radical prostatectomy requires extensive learning; approximately 40 cases are needed to master this technique. In contrast, the learning of robotic prostatectomy seems to be more intuitive and less demanding. Wood and Woolf compared 10 robotic prostatectomies with 10 laparoscopic prostatectomies, all performed by the same surgeon, who is an experienced upper urinary tract laparoscopist.[20] Despite this surgeon's large amount of laparoscopic experience, the mean operative time was on average 145 minutes less for robotic than for laparoscopic prostatectomy.

The estimated blood loss was comparable (< 500 cc), and there were two conversions (to RRP) in each group, but no major complications occurred. The authors' group[1] performed 48 laparoscopic radical prostatectomies and 50 robot-assisted prostatectomies within a 12-month period. The preoperative and intraoperative demographical variables were comparable in both groups as were the operative times, changes in hemoglobin concentrations, durations of hospitalization, positive margin rates, and overall complication rates. All measured clinical and pathologic parameters were comparable to the best laparoscopic radical prostatectomy results reported in the literature.[1]

Author's Conclusions

Robotic prostatectomy is a safe, effective and reproducible technique for removing the prostate. In most patients, it can be performed within one and a half to two hours with minimal blood loss and few complications. The procedure incorporates principles of both laparoscopic and open radical prostatectomy. The patients enjoy benefits of surgical treatment in the setting of less invasion, minimal pain, limited blood loss and early functional and overall recovery.

Selected References Cited By Authors:

1. Menon M, Shrivastava A, Tewari A, Sarle R, Hemal A, Peabody JO, Vallancien G: Laparoscopic and robot assisted radical prostatectomy: establishment of a structured program and preliminary analysis of outcomes. J Urol. 2002 sep;168(3):945-9.

2. Stoianovici D: Robotic surgery. Worl J Urol, 18: 289, 2000.

3. Cadeddu JA, Stoianovici D, Kavoussi LR: Robotic surgery in urology. Urol Clin North Am, 25: 75, 1998.

4. Hubert J: Robotic pyeloplasty. Curr Urol Rep, 4: 124, 2003.

5. Menon M, Shrivastava A, Sarle R et al: Vattikuti Institute Prostatectomy: a single-team experience of 100 cases. J Endourol, 17: 785, 2003.

6. Leak B, Wei JT, Gabel, M et al: Relevant patient and tumor considerations for early prostate cancer treatment. Semin Urol Oncol, 20: 39, 2002.

7. Tewari A, Menon M, Peabody J et al: An anatomic map to assist identification of the neurovascular bundle during laparoscopic radical prostatectomy. New Delhi: B.I. Churchill Livingstone, pp. 297-304, 2002.

8. Tewari A, Peabody J, Sarle R et al: Technique of da vinci robot-assisted anatomic radical prostatectomy. Urology, 60: 569, 2002.

9. Tewari A, Menon M: Vattikuti institute prostatectomy: surgical technique and current results. Curr Urol Rep, 4(2):119-23, 2003.

10. Tewari A, Menon M, Peabody J et al: An operative and anatomic study to help in nerve sparing during laparoscopic and robotic radical prostatectomy. Eur Urol 43:444-54, 2003.

11. Tewari A, Srivasatava A, Menon M: A prospective comparison of radical retropubic and robot-assisted prostatectomy: experience in one institution. BJU Int, 92: 205, 2003.

12. Tewari A, Peabody JO, Fischer M et al: An operative and anatomic study to help in nerve sparing during laparoscopic and robotic radical prostatectomy. Eur Urol, 43: 444, 2003.

13. Menon M, Tewari A, Baize B et al: A prospective comparison of robot-assisted anatomic prostatectomy and conventional radical retropubic prostatectomy: the Vattikuti Urology Institute experience. Urology 60:864-8, 2002.

14. Menon M, Tewari A, Baize B et al: Prospective comparison of radical retropubic prostatectomy and robot-assisted anatomic prostatectomy: the Vattikuti Urology Institute experience. Urology, 60: 864, 2002.

15. Menon M, Tewari A, Peabody J: Technique of Vattikuti Institute Prostatectomy. J. Urol.: in press, 2002.

16. Menon M, Tewari A, Peabody J: Vattikuti Institute prostatectomy: technique. J Urol, 169: 2289, 2003.

17. Tewari A, Johnson CC, Divine G et al: Long-term survival probability in men with clinically localized prostate cancer: a case-control, propensity modeling study stratified by race, age, treatment and comorbidities. J Urol, 171: 1513, 2004.

18. Menon M, Tewari A: Robotic radical prostatectomy and the Vattikuti Urology Institute technique: an interim analysis of results and technical points. Urology, 61: 15, 2003.

19. Diefenbach MA, Dorsey J, Uzzo RG et al: Decision-making strategies for patients with localized prostate cancer. Semin Urol Oncol, 20: 55, 2002.

20. Wood DP, Wolf JS: Oncology rather than laparoscopy surgical experience is more important in learning to perform a robotassisted laparoscopic radical prostatectomy. J Urol. 2004; 171(4 Suppl, Abstract 813): 215.

....

NOTE: These papers and studies are only a sampling of the various publications that explain the tremendous advancements in surgical treatment methods for prostate cancer. The last paper that is provided here, comes from the Prostate Cancer Research Institute, a non-profit research center located in southern California.

According to their website, The Prostate Cancer Research Institute (PCRI) was founded in 1996 by medical oncologists Stephen B. Strum and Mark C. Scholz, with support from the Daniel Freeman Hospital Foundation in Southern California. According to PCRI, Dr. Strum and Dr. Scholz are internationally recognized prostate cancer specialists. From the PCRI website:

> "...the objective of PCRI is to educate patients and their families about prostate cancer. This includes new advances in diagnosis, staging, treatments and available resources. PCRI believes that a patient who understands his disease and treatment is empowered to communicate more effectively with his physicians and obtain a better outcome. PCRI intends to use all available communication tools to accomplish this most important objective."

Prostate Cancer 2.0 objectives are to present balanced and accurate information about the treatment options that are available for prostate cancer, with a minimum of unproven and undocumented accolades not supported by research and referred Journal papers. Those goals appear to be consistent with the mission statement goals of PCRI and, therefore, the following paper is provided here as one of the best explanations for what the robotic-assisted procedure is and what its capability has to offer. It is written in understandable 'lay' language while also utilizing studies data taken from clinical and hospital settings, where real-world prostate cancer patients are treated.

The reader is directed to the PCRI website to view the complete paper with all its accompanying diagrams, tables, pictures, and even video explanations for further clarity.

Major Studies Underway

There is a major Department of Defense (DOD) research effort under way called the Prostate Cancer Research Program (PCRP) that was established in 1997 to promote innovative research focused on *eradicating* prostate cancer. So far a total of $1.05 Billion had been appropriated (by DOD) through FY2011, to that effort. Since that first year, Two hundred sixty proposals resulted in 26 projects being awarded to 54 researchers who are in collaborative partnership efforts intended to 'synergisticlly achieve results not possible for individual research investigators by themselves..." (PCRP's words).

So far, these projects have not resulted in any new technologies or treatment methodologies that have met the goal that DOE's Congressionally Directed Medical Programs Group envisioned, although incremental progress has been shown in the use of robotic surgical techniques. For some, that may justify the investment, but the newest round of awards for FY2011 still has the intent (*) to ***"significantly accelerate advances in prostate cancer research to support the PCRP vision of conquering prostate cancer..."***

(*) *Author's Note: As of May 2012, reports on research results from these DOD-sponsored projects were not yet available, so whether or not there has been 'significant acceleration advances (to benefit PC patient's) is still a question.*

For the diagnosed PC sufferer, this may only serve notice that your government is, indeed, concerned about prostate cancer and wants to spend taxpayer monies to eradicate it by synergistically accelerating the research (and thus, the methodologies for curing the disease), but the results of this expenditure so far, will not help you find the treatment that will eradicate YOUR cancer. After 14 years of 26 ongoing research projects, there is no evidence that PC cures have been "accelerated" or will be forthcoming any time soon.

If you are interested in pursuing this research, you can query the DOD's Congressionally Directed Medical Research Program...but, don't expect a rapid reply or silver bullet to be forthcoming any time soon---but do know, your government is here to help you!

"IF YOU HAVE BEEN DIAGNOSED WITH CANCER (ANY CANCER... NOT *ONLY* PROSTATE CANCER, YOU ABSOLUTELY *MUST* SEEK MORE THAN ONE MEDICAL OPINION ABOUT YOUR TREATMENT OPTIONS! AND, YOU ABSOLUTELY *MUST* SEEK OPINIONS FROM DIFFERENT TREATMENT SPECIALISTS: SURGERY, RADIATION, CRYOGENICS, ROBOTICS SURGERY; ETC."

CHAPTER FIVE

In this chapter, you will learn about...

Rethinking Treatment Options: The Mayo Clinic Study

When should men start PSA screening?

Discussing Cancer Screening With Doctors

INTRODUCTION

This is a short chapter to review some issues that have been discussed in greater detail in other chapters. Many people have been aware of the wonderful and successful work done at the Mayo Clinic in Rochester, Minnesota in so many other areas (other than PC treatment) so I thought it important to give you their general thinking when it comes to PC treatment options. In addition, because I have presumed that you have already been diagnosed (and, thus, would not be thinking about whether or not to have a PSA exam), you might still want to know what the medical community is recently saying about the pros and cons of having that test done, so there is a section in this chapter that discusses that.

MAYO CLINIC STUDIES: Rethinking Radiation Treatment Options

A Mayo Clinic study by Dr. O.K. McDonald and Dr. Steven Schild (Mayo Clinic, 2003), of men who have had a reoccurrence of cancer after a prostatectomy was conducted in Scottsdale, Arizona focused on men whose PSA levels rose after surgery (ie, radical prostatectomy), up to five years later. The results showed, among other things, that 20% of men whose prostates were removed had their PSA levels rise, indicating that cancer has come back.

In the Mayo study, 60 men with elevated PSA levels were given radiation treatments over seven weeks at the site where the prostate was removed. They followed the treated men and after 5 years, half the men treated with radiation are free of cancer, with those men who received higher radiation doses doing better than those treated with lower doses.

In discussing the conclusions of the study at the Chicago meeting of the American Society of Clinical Oncology (May, 2003), Dr. Schild noted that when primary care providers and urologists send someone for radiation treatment, it's better to send them earlier than later. *"Now that we know that men who have a return of cancer after a prostatectomy should be treated with higher dosages of radiation to improve chances for a cure."*

The priority treatment at Mayo Clinic has historically been radical prostatectamy for most cancer patients, no matter what Gleason Scores indicate. It appears, on the basis of this study, the Mayo Clinic oncologists, urologists, and prostate specialists are now taking a second look at that policy, perhaps to looking at brachytherapy and Electron Beam treatment before recommending radical prostatectomy as the first priority.

PSA SCREENING: What age to start?

It has been shown that GP's are beginning to take more seriously the DRE in routine physical exams. There is a sharper awareness in the general medical community that PSA results should be *routinely* requested in blood work for physical examinations, although there is some evidence that insurance companies are balking at paying for this test in men under the age of 50 without justification on a case by case basis.

There is also a growing concern, among general practicioners at least, that men who have symptoms of prostate problems should be more closely observed and followed and sent to urologists for evaluation even when PSA results are low. Generally, the symptoms most often cited are BPH or routine physical exam results that night-time visits to the bathroom are becoming an issue, seem to be triggering more GP concern than when the First Edition surveys were conducted. Of course, it is also unclear if the impetus for this follow-up is concern might be about potential liability and malpractice or even if the general awareness of the medical community that younger and younger men are having prostate 'symptoms' that GPs are taking note about. But, the medical community in general has become more sensitive to cancer as more and more work has been done on the diagnostic side of medicine. The results are more important for men: more attention is now being focused on prostate cancer than at anytime in history.

The consensus of doctors involved in men's health now appears to be directed toward taking a hard look at PSA results on physical exams that are otherwise routine. The picture we need to paint now is that men of every age should be as knowledgeable about what PSA means (i.e. how good an indicator it is or is not). If this book accomplishes nothing else, that should be one issue that gets clearly defined: PSA is the best indicator ***at this point in time*** (emphasis added!) of the potential for prostate cancer to be present. It is not, however, infallible and numerical values assigned to it are debated by specialists across the medical professions. Is a result of 2.9 different from 2.5? Should you be concerned if PSA results are greater than 3.0 or 4.0? the actual hard and fast "number" is not something physicians, especially general practicioners, agree on so why should a man be expected to understand what to do when such results are reported?

Thus, what is important to know is, that there *should* be follow-up if the numerical value consistently rises, from blood tests taken 3 or 4 times over as many months. That '*trend*' rise indicates the possibility that something is going on and a urologist needs to evaluate your options, usually meaning that a biopsy should be performed---but not always.

Whether or not a biopsy should be conducted under that circumstance is, of course, a matter of agreement between a man and his doctor. Second opinions are encouraged to get consensus but, generally a rising PSA (with values greater than 3.5) probably should result in a biopsy. Even then, understand the biopsy procedure and the risks that procedure subjects you to before selecting the doctor to conduct it. (Read Chapters One and Three again!)

Some clinics and prostate doctors look at the PSA results in age increments. For instance, for men who have PSA results less than 3.0, most will say there's nothing to worry about but to re-test in 2 to 6 months to see if it increases or remains relatively unchanged. For men bracketed in the age group 40 to 50, some will say a PSA of less than 3.0 is OK while, for men age 50 to 60 they might say a PSA score of up to 4.0 is OK. For men 50 to 60, they might say a PSA up to 5.0 is OK and for men 60 to 70, they might say a PSA of up to 6.0 would be OK, prescribing "watch and wait" for each of those age brackets and PSA scores. For men over 70, they may say "don't worry until the PSA reaches greater than, say, 6.5 and, even then, re-testing every 3 months to see if there is a trend might be the prognosis.

Advice: Consult Health Practicioners

Drugs, PSAs, and BPH

Remember, in an earlier discussion, about Finasteride (Proscar) studies in 2003/4 that were showing that BPH sufferers who used preventative hormonal therapy might reduce the risk that they would have prostate cancer later on? The UC-Berkeley Wellness Letter of September, 2008, reported that "…a long awaited Federal study…" ---(which was *not* specified so we don't know if the study was peer reviewed or even how the study was conducted or if it was the same study from 2003 that had just concluded)---"found that a drug widely used to treat urinary symptoms caused by prostate enlargement (BPH) had been found to reduce the ***risk*** of prostate cancer in men over age 55 by 25%." The Letter went on to say that, "… Finasteride, brand named Proscar and available in generic form with a prescription), is thought to inhibit the conversion of testosterone to dihydrotestosterone which is a hormone that can cause prostate growth as well as encourage prostate cancer cell growth and, by the way, hair loss."

But here is the important information gleaned from the Wellness Letter: The study, called the Prostate Cancer Prevention Trial (PCPT), concluded that while the drug reduced the risk of ***insignificant*** cancers (what are insignificant cancers, you ask? The study doesn't explain that), it seemed to increase the risk of more aggressive types. This led to further analyses of the PCPT research using more thorough and complete data (i.e. remember the adage that statistics lie and liars use statistics; highlighting (manipulating?) the numbers in such ways as to get the outcomes they want might apply here---have shown that ultimately "…the initial findings about finasteride was misleading and that men taking the drug had a lower rate of ALL types of prostate cancer, including the aggressive ones."

Not only does the drug appear to prevent or slow the *development* of cancer, but by shrinking the prostate, it may also make it easier to detect tumors that do develop.

But, before the medical community will tout this therapy as the magic elixir for prostate cancer (risk) reduction to be prescribed for *ALL* men before any symptoms are observed, there are a lot of questions to be answered. The usual side effects of hormone therapy have already been observed in patients that have been taking Finasteride for BPH; such side effects include erectile dysfunction and, less often, breast growth. And no one knows what side effects might manifest for men who take the drug as a preventive measure who have normal prostates and no BPH symptoms---studies need to be done on men that are taking the drug for hair growth, usually Propecia (although it contains 1/5th the dose that is used to treat BPH), to get a large enough sample to make statistical inferences possible. This would also include the under-40 or 50 age men who are least likely to have BPH symptoms.

In addition to these studies in the early 2000's showing that BPH treatment drugs have promise as a treatment that may slow the progressive growth of PC tumors in diagnosed men, the follow-up studies that were given preliminary results in Chapter Three, show that Avodart actually produced good results in low-risk (i.e. is that the same as 'insignificant' cancer cells) PC sufferers. What those studies didn't discuss, however, is what the side-effects (or after-effects) of treatment with Avodart are: with most hormonal drugs, men will immediately suffer ED and perhaps, some of the other side effects like stimulated breast growth. Of course, these would seem to be a small price to pay if the alternative was rapid and untreatable cancer cell growth.

And, there are other drugs called dutasteride (brand named Avodart) that are being studied as a cancer preventive in high-risk men---men who have a family history or African-American men fall in the high-risk category. These studies will take longer, of course, so men in the high risk category, Avodart should not be viewed as their therapy which will automatically lower their risks for getting prostate cancer---the data is not there yet to support this contention.

Not A Silver Bullet

It does, however, cause some further concerns: if the administration of Finasteride (or Proscar or Propecia or any other hormone deprivation therapy) results in a lowering of PSA, in general, will that give men a false sense of security and keep them thinking they may OK when, the lowering of the PSA "number" does not necessarily mean the cancer cells are not present but, rather, there has been some type of interaction with the antigen (the Prostate <u>*Specific*</u> Antigen that the "number" represents) which somehow keeps it from being accurately 'extracted' in the blood test.

For the man who has already been biopsied and *knows* he has prostate cancer, all of this news about preventative drug therapies is merely interesting and academic. You have been diagnosed and your needs are now, 1.) how to I treat my cancer and 2.) what should you shoud do first? That is what this second edition of <u>***Prostate Cancer 2.0***</u> is about: your options for successfully eliminating cancer cells in your prostate.

PSA: What The *Numbers* Represent

As discussed above in the hormone therapy studies, PSA as an indicator for presence of cancer cells in the prostate is, at best, just one way that doctors look for data they can use for diagnostics. Thus, it is not our recommendation to interpret PSA *numbers* by a sliding scale in age brackets. Research findings for this Edition 2.0, seems to show consistent agreement with the idea that PSA scores greater than 3.0 ng per milliliter for *any* age should be followed with re-testing over a six month period. The exception might be for men over age 70 or 75, where higher PSA scores might require retesting only every 6 months to see if a trend is developing. Even then, it may be questionable to recommend "treatment" for the man who has other, more serious, medical conditions. Again, this is the place for men to get second and third opinions before deciding to take any sort of action.

The fact that more and more doctors are concerned about accurately communicating the pros and cons of prostate health is supported in the literature. More clinics and hospitals are making prostate information available now than ever before. But, doctors who treat and diagnose prostate problems are not any more forthcoming than they ever have been, and men need to understand how to get answers *before* they decide on a specific treatment regime, especially where cancer has been diagnosed. There is a reason why those commercials on TV touting drugs for BPH (like Flomax and Flonase) tell you to always *"ask your doctor, since only s/he can tell you if your symptoms are cancer or not...).* Just be aware that doctors will only be as detailed as they need to be to put the decision making responsibility on your shoulders---or, more accurately, on your prostate ---you will have to ask questions---the ***RIGHT*** questions---to make an informed decision about what treatment is best for you.

That is why, this book intentionally repeats the admonishment in every chapter: get a second, third, and even a fourth opinion---visit both urologists and oncologists who practice prostate-specific medicine. The treatment you choose will have profound effects on your body for the rest of your life so do not ever approach the treatment decision lightly.

DISCUSSING CANCER SCREENING WITH DOCTORS

Because there is a renewed emphasis within the medical community on making sure that prostate cancer is diagnosed in its earliest stages, there are differing opinions on what the diagnostic steps should be. For patients who come to the GP with symptoms, there is an almost universal tendency for recommending follow-up with a urologist. (Here is where the 'communications' begin to break down, for the patient and we talk about that problem here). For the routine physical exam that shows PSA abnormalities or DRE deviation of the prostate gland, we find that whatever recommendation is made to the patient is related to how old the examining physician is and how long he or she has been in practice! Most of this 'finding' is based on anecdotal or heresay from conversations with patients, but the information is valuable for the newly concerned man going for recommendations.

INFORMATION SOURCES

The advent of the World Wide Web (Internet) has provided anyone who has access to a computer or an iPhone anywhere in the world, with access to data and information that was never before possible. Gone are the days when the only way to learn about an unfamiliar topic or subject was to go to a city or college library, use the card catalog and/or consult the librarian to conduct a research of the literature that took days or even weeks. Even then, obtaining even half of the information requested was hit or miss, depending upon how capable the research assistant was and how big the library capability was to "cover the globe."

Today, there are internet access kiosks at coffee shops and in the smallest of town libraries and easy "how to" guides to make a novice computer hacker an expert at finding information. For purposes of this book, we have included some of the sites (i.e. even this list will lead to more sites that are linked to these) that may prove useful to the interested researcher specific to Prostate Cancer information.

One note of caution: the internet sites come and go with more being added daily to the World Wide Web. Therefore, the sites noted in this book are not a comprehensive list. So, when (and if) you go the internet, you can query sites like, "www.ask.com" or "www.google.com" by searching for the key words, such as "brachytherapy" or "prostate" or any combination of words related to the topic. What those sites will do is "connect" you to sites that have those words or phrases as a partial subject for their site. But, after searching for a while, you will find that you begin to get repeated site names more and more frequently as they seem to "link together." Thus, at that point, you will probably want to begin getting into the sites that you think give you the information you are looking for, and conclude your mission of searching for new sites.

In total, however, you will find conflicting advice and you will need to think for yourself, sound out your thoughts with your doctor(s) , and talk to other men who have the same problem to be sure you can make decisions about your own situation. The key is, however, BE INFORMED and don't accept ONE opinion from ONE doctor. It's *your* prostate! Its *your* health! And, its *your* responsibility to yourself to get the best advice and information you can.

Men of all ages: Take Charge!

Summarizing this chapter with an admonishment (risking redundancy): men need to be better informed about their prostate health and recommend that they seek out every source of information they can find. This would be essential not only for men who are just beginning to have prostate symptoms but, as well, for men who have never had reason to be concerned. The message is this: get a PSA every year, together with an annual physical exam, starting at age 40!

It has become "popular" for journalists who write for various health organizations to eschew the value of screening for PC, particularly the value of getting a PSA with your physical exam every year. Somehow, the seed of disillusionment has been planted by the medical community that prostate cancer is not easily diagnosed by a simple blood test---somehow, men are over reacting when they get the news that their PSA results are "high" (i.e. they question if we really know what "high" means in the first place)---and that sending them off to get a biopsy on the flimsy evidence that the PSA screening test provides somehow subjects them to risks that outweigh the benefit of knowing.

Gary Schwitzer, a health journalist and publisher of HealthNewsReview.org provides a good example of this kind of this rhetoric in his February 2011 Consumer Reports on Health (One Minute Consult), titled *News On Screenings*:

"What Could Be The Harm Of A Screening Test?

> Schwitzer's Ans: Take the PSA blood test for prostate cancer: People ask, "why wouldn't I roll up my sleeve for this test?" Well, many men die with prostate cancer silently inside them, not from it. We don't really know the benefit of treating the early cancers we find from that blood test, but we do know that treatment may have many side effects, such as incontinence or impotence. Or take the recent trial of CT scans to screen for early lung cancers. One in four people who got the scans had a "positive" result that turned out not to be lung cancer at all. You would have to screen 300 people---and remember, this study only looked at people who were already at high risk for lung cancer because of a history of heavy smiling----to extend the life of one person. The other 299 experienced harm, ranging from having to pay the cost of the test on up through worry, more radiation, and biopsies for false negatives.

How Can People Decide Whether They Should Get A Screening Test?

> Schwitzer's Ans: The U.S. Preventative Services Task Force provides great detail on the evidence for and against screening tests. If your doctor recommends a test, ask what happens if you get a positive result. If you read a news report about a screening test that only talks about benefits and not harms, you should question the source because you are probably getting incomplete picture of the trade-offs involved. Also, find out whether the test is for the whole population or just for people at high risk, for example, because their family members died of the disease. If we confuse the two, we'll confuse the trade-off of harms and benefits."

While this line of reasoning is being parroted by a few doctors, it is being endorsed mostly by so-called health reporters across a wide spectrum of popular media and there are just not a lot of studies or clinical results that support this kind of logic. Obviously, it is the conclusion of PC Edition 2.0 that the best way men can know if PC is present is by PSA screening tests every year. It is, in fact, the ONLY way to catch it in the early stages when we can have options for treating it and, subsequently, living a healthy life!

The observation that the cost for a physical exam, even if you must pay for it out of pocket, is cheap when compared with finding a problem when its too late to treat it. Prostate Cancer is treatable and curable, if it is diagnosed in the early stages. Ordinary physical examinations which include a PSA blood screen will pay dividends in the cost-benefit analysis.

The choices you have if and when results show cause for concern are expanding every day for most men's diseases, and especially in cancers of the prostate and colon, early diagnosis is essential to treatment choice options that lead to living a long and healthy life. In order to do this right, men absolutely ***MUST*** be proactive and take charge of their physical conditions. Take yearly exams; develop a good rapport with your GP, and communicate! Its *your* life – live it!

"IF YOU HAVE BEEN DIAGNOSED WITH CANCER (ANY CANCER...) NOT JUST PROSTATE CANCER, YOU ABSOLUTELY *MUST* SEEK MORE THAN ONE MEDICAL OPINION ABOUT YOUR TREATMENT OPTIONS! AND, YOU ABSOLUTELY *MUST* SEEK OPINIONS FROM DIFFERENT TREATMENT SPECIALISTS: SURGERY, RADIATION, CRYOGENICS, ROBOTICS SURGERY; ETC."

CHAPTER SIX

In this chapter, you will learn about....

PREVENTION AND NUTRITION

DO's AND DON'T DO's: A Brief Review of Food Choices

FOODS AND SCIENCE

LIFESTYLE CHOICES: Living A Healthy Life

Alternative Medicine and Treatment Techniques

Once Again: Get More Than One Opinion

DON'T ASK; DON'T TELL

Prevention And Alternative Medicine

LOOKING FOR SCIENCE: Ask The Scientists!

VITAMINS AND HERBS: Not A Substitute

SUMMARIZING SCIENCE: Drugs Are *Really* Big Business!

ALTERNATIVE THERAPIES FROM OTHER CANCERS: The Case For Laetrile

INTRODUCTION

Prevention has become a much used and abused word in medicine today. But, it really is the best way to ensure that people live a lifestyle today that recognizes that what they eat and how they exercise (or don't), can have significant benefits in the prevention of disease in the future. Some physicians believe that this is the only way, in fact, to give the body the best opportunity to prevent diseases, including cancer, from starting. Statistics on life and death in the 21st century appear to bear that out: In 1900, the average baby born could expect to live 47.3 years while, in 2000, life expectancy had risen to 76.9 years. According to the National Center for Health

Statistics (September, 2002), drops in death rates at every stage of life and for most diseases, is occurring nationwide. Even with the introduction of killer diseases like AIDS, preventative life style choices such as not smoking and preventative medical intervention (i.e. technology), has had a dramatic effect on increased life expectancy.

Interestingly, mortality among adults ages 45 to 64 fell by nearly 50 percent between 1950 and 2000, including drops in heart disease, stroke and injury. But, cancer is still the leading cause of death in this group, although the rates rose until 1980 when they began to drop slowly. Just as puzzling, however, is the fact that, while cancer rates have been falling since 1980, prostate cancer rates have risen over that same period. Thus, statistics must always be compared and applied with a note of caution: Prostate cancer is still on the rise and men need to understand what their risk factors are, *before* making life style choices.

The word, '*disease*,' after all is made up of two terms: 'dis' and 'ease' so that the noun, 'disease' can virtually be used to describe a plethora of maladies. That includes 'cancer' of course, and any discussion of cancer should include the ways we believe that 'prevention' of the disease can, at least, be enhanced.

In this discussion, we recognize that the jury is still out on what eating properly and exercising regularly actually contributes to *prevention*, particularly as it applies to cancer prevention. In the case of prostate cancer, this is even more obscure because little is yet known about what causes cancer cells to suddenly begin multiplying in the gland. If we knew, we might be able to say what 'preventative' measures are absolutely certain to prevent prostate cancer. But, we don't know. Thus, in this chapter, we explore what medical and preventative measures we believe will provide better circumstances for prevention of cancer (both general cancer in the body, as well as prostate cancer specifically).

We also are concerned with the man who already knows he has prostate cancer---or, perhaps, other cancer elsewhere. But, primarily the information here is for the man who is either being treated for, or has been treated for prostate cancer: what does the literature have to say about alternative medicine and herbs, as it relates to prostate cancer?

Of course, it will be controversial once more, whenever the term ***'alternative medicine'*** is used. But, such controversy is healthy and we encourage discussion and debate on the use of alternative therapies. And, it is vitally important that we provide you with as much information as possible on the ways in which you might live a healthy and long life.

Do's and Don't Do's: A Brief Review of Food Choices

Nutritionists and herbalists have a plethora of "foods" that have been promoted over the years for making up a healthy diet. Unfortunately, each practicioner seems to have favorite "*foods*" they like or dislike and they are not all in agreement. In our concern to find *'science-based'* recommendations for this text, we have provided only those **cancer-avoidance** 'foods' which have some scientifically validated data behind them.

As noted in the Introduction to this text, we still don't know what triggers prostate cancer tumors to grow so we cannot say with certainty, which 'foods' to eat or to avoid, to prevent prostate cancer. In fact, no one really knows for sure if food, in fact, has anything at all to do with prostate cancer. But, there have recently begun to be more peer reviewed studies being conducted in well respected universities and by the National Cancer Institute that, while "prospective" in nature (i.e. meaning they are studies that record what people *say* they eat and then follow them for years to see who gets sick and who doesn't) linking the consumption of well-done meat and poultry with an increased risk of prostate cancer.

Being 'prospective' studies that use questionnaires that are answered by the 'subjects' themselves, one peer reviewer noted that one of the NCI's studies was subject to a fair bit of imprecision that researchers needed to evaluate when drawing conclusions. But, generally, evidence seems to be building that well done meat (*any* meat: pork, chicken, beef) might increase the risk of several kinds of cancer, prostate cancer being just one type that was studied. The problem here is, for poultry at least, about 40% of raw poultry has been found to contain salmonella bacteria and it is highly recommended that ALL poultry be cooked thoroughly, at high temperatures, in order to kill the salmonella bacteria, before serving. Thus, it is prudent to weigh the risks: prevention of cancer vs. food poisoning---but, the evidence for linking well done meat to cancer is weak, so it is probably best to over-cook poultry and deal with other preventative measures for the increased risk that cancer might be linked to over-cooked meat.

Here are some examples: in a study that was published in *Cancer Epidemiology* (2008), of 23,000 U.S. agricultural workers, NCI researchers found that men who ate the most well done or very well done meat and poultry (about 20 ounces a week) were twice as likely to be diagnosed with advanced prostate cancer as men who ate the least (or 4 ounces or less per week) meat that was well done.

In a study of 29,000 U.S. men, those who ate the most very well done meat and poultry---at least 2 ½ ounces a week---were 70% more likely to be diagnosed with prostate cancer than those who ate none. This particular study only looked at men who said they ate meat *very* well done, and not at respondents who said they ate meat (only) well done or *less* well done than *very* well done. Still, this result does suggest a pretty high rate of positive results for prostate cancer for men who preferred their meat to be well cooked.

The September 2008 Nutrition Action Healthletter which reported these NCI study results noted that "a preference for well done meat might be one reason why African-American men have the highest rates of prostate cancer in the world. Black American men consume two to three times more (well cooked) meat than white American men, according to Lawrence Livermore scientists who peer reviewed the NCI studies...." But, this is only conjecture and not a "result" that comes from this study---no one yet knows why black men have a higher incidence of prostate cancer, and this study didn't show this linkage.

Lawrence Livermore scientist and researcher Garrett Keating had this to say about the possible implications for Black men: *"A light went on* (and) *we thought maybe this would explain their high rates of prostate cancer."*

Personally, I wouldn't put much faith on one study that assumes people have filled out a questionnaire knowing the difference between 'well cooked' and very well cooked meat to make such blanket judgments that they've found *the* reason why the rate of prostate cancer in African-American men is so much higher than in Caucasian men---but, the study certainly adds data to the mounting evidence that high heterocyclic amine (HCA) levels are created in meat, poultry, and fish by high-heat in cooking---about 20 different HCAs have been isolated in cooked meat and at least one has been found to cause colon, breast and prostate tumors in lab animals. Nonetheless, the studies are worth considering when we are trying to find reasons for why prostate cancer occurs in some men and not in others.

Since 2001, Keating and his colleagues have been monitoring about 400 African-American men in their 50s, 60s, and 70s in Oakland California and have seen that those who consume the most meat and poultry that (they say is well cooked or very well cooked), have very high PSA levels of 20 or higher, than those who eat the least meats, in general. So, for African-American men, the reduction of meat and poultry in the diet in general and the reduction of well cooked or very well cooked meat and poultry specifically would seem to be prudent across the board.

Again, understanding that there might be a link between men who eat highly cooked meat or poultry and prostate cancer becomes merely interesting for the man who has already been diagnosed with cancer. What man cares why he got the disease when he's facing choices for how to get rid of it and go on living a healthy and productive life? So, we digress---but for the future, look for a lot more studies on the association of foods we consume and prostate cancer.

Foods Before and After Prostate Cancer

Nutritional science and herbal practice over the past 3000 years has given us a fairly good idea of what 'foods' are more healthy and what 'foods' generally cause more morbidity in the general population. It is this body of 'food' *science* that we take our recommendations from and hope you will experiment with your own 'recipes' to find out what works best for *your* body.

As noted before, Dr. Larry Clapp (Prostate Health in 90 Days, 2000), has written and published widely about the *correct* (*his* opinion) foods for both general health and cancer prevention. He notes that most Americans don't even come close to eating a healthy diet, preferring the four food groups beginning with the letter, 'f', instead: *fried* food, *fast* food, *frozen* food, and *fun* food (candy). (pp 111).

As our life styles have evolved into hectic scheduling marathons, family mealtime has been sacrificed in the interest of stuffing in before and after school activities, weekend sports and music lessons, and road trips to see or play activities that almost demand fast food stops instead of home-cooked meals. It may be that, if we did nothing else in the way of deciding what 'foods' we should and shouldn't be eating, we could have a great impact on reducing prostate (and other) cancer simply by giving up all those hectic and stressful activities that have taken us away from family meals at home. No one, however, has studied this possibility so we are left with speculating about what foods, given our hectic life style choices, should and shouldn't be in our diet.

The Linus Pauling Institute Cancer Research

Dr. Emily Ho is a research scientist at the Linus Pauling Institute at Oregon State University in Corvallis, Oregon. She has been conducting studies on essential minerals and their impact on cancer in mice. One of her studies focused on zinc in the prostate, and its use as a preventative therapy or, as treatment for prostate cancer. Here's a partial interview that was published in the LPI Research Newsletter in Fall 2008:

Q. You have done a lot of work with zinc and prostate cancer using cell cultures. What have you found?

A. The prostate has the highest concentration of zinc of all the soft tissues in the body—bone is the only other tissue that has more zinc. The prostate accumulates zinc, but we don't know why. In prostate cancer, the zinc levels dramatically drop dose-dependently with disease progression. We want to understand these phenomena better.

Q. Do zinc levels decline with age in men?

A. We're looking into that. As I mentioned, zinc status in humans is really difficult to assess, but there is some evidence that zinc levels decrease with age. We think that absorption may change with age. Older people eat less, and they are not able to absorb as much zinc. Most of the studies have been done in women. If you give zinc supplements to young women and older women, plasma zinc levels will increase in the young but not in the older women. With men, it doesn't look like zinc supplementation is going to be a cure for prostate cancer. We haven't seen much effect of zinc in decreasing cancer in our rodent studies, but we have found that low zinc levels cause problems in the prostate with respect to oxidative stress, DNA damage, and mutations that could increase the risk for cancer.

Q. Does zinc have any effect on prostate cancer malignancy?

A. The more aggressive cancers seem to have less zinc. One problem is that the cancer cells have adapted to a low zinc status, so if you give zinc, they are more resistant. We have been a little bit disappointed with the fact that once you have cancer, zinc doesn't help much. On the other hand, zinc may play an important role in preventing prostate cancer.

Q. What are the most effective dietary strategies to protect against prostate cancer?

A. There's no magic bullet, but consumption of fruits and vegetables is associated with decreased risk. Our research suggests that cruciferous vegetables might be helpful. People in Asia have a very low incidence of prostate cancer, but when they move to the United States, it dramatically increases because of dietary changes. Also, there has been a low prostate cancer risk in China, but as they become more industrialized, there is a slow but steady increase in prostate cancer. Eating a lot of fat or red meat seems to increase the risk. Obesity is a risk factor for prostate cancer partly because of its associated inflammation and hormones that may change with increased adiposity.

ZINC AND HUMAN DEFICIENCY

Zinc is an essential micronutrient that is present in virtually all cells in the body. The primary functions of zinc in biological systems can be categorized as catalytic, structural, and regulatory, which is to say that it is required for the formation and stabilization of protein structure and is essential for the activity of more than 300 enzymes. The connection between zinc deficiency and cancer has been suggested by several large epidemiological, observational cohort studies that have confirmed that the deficiency response is an impaired DNA integrity which increases or makes cells susceptible to abnormal growth.

Since it is well understood that DNA damage can occur by numerous agents such as ionizing radiation, ultraviolet light, reactive oxygen species, ethidium bromide, and food-borne carcinogens like polycyclic aromatic hydrocarbons and hetrocyclic amines---as well as deficiencies of vitamin C, vitamin E, iron, and, of course, zinc---accumulation of DNA mutations is an essential event in cancer initiation, promotion, and progression.

During the promotion stage, initiated cells start to grow and differentiate rapidly and accumulate DNA mutations, resulting in changes in cell behavior. In the progression stage, cancer cells grow aggressively resulting the appearance of a small tumor. At this stage, studies have shown that zinc depletion in cells increase DNA damage, although the effects of zinc deficiency on DNA integrity in cells in the body are still unclear.

In other studies in the LPI lab, the focus is on zinc depletion on DNA integrity in vivo where the research intends to try to understand the mechanisms of these effects. So far, the in vivo studies where marginal zinc depletion was shown to cause DNA strand breaks in the peripheral blood cells of rats, the damage was reversible and could be reduced to normal levels by zinc repletion. Similar effects were observed in human subjects, indicating that zinc is also essential for maintaining DNA integrity in humans.

Of course, replication of DNA cells requires that those cells be present in the particular organ---in this case, the prostate gland---in order that cells could, in fact, be repaired by bringing the zinc levels back through some type of supplement routine. If results of these in vivo studies are to show success in repairing DNA cells that are involved in cancer propagation, those cells would be inside the prostate gland *only* if the gland had not been surgically removed prior to the administration of zinc supplements. So far, that part of the study has yet to be completed.

For the concerned man who wants to use supplements as a preventative measure, this in vivo study would seem to offer good evidence that zinc supplements are a *potential* way to lower the risk for prostate cancer, although there is little proof yet available that this single vitamin is the silver bullet for prostate cancer propagation.

It is worth noting that, in rat studies conducted at the LPI, "a combination of both marginal zinc deficiency and high intensity chronic exercise...markedly increased DNA damage in the prostate...(but) only in the dorsolateral---not the ventral---lobes of the prostate." And, according to LPI scientists, about 70% of human prostate cancers are found in the human prostate area equivalent to the rat dorsolateral lobe, and that is the lobe that is most sensitive to marginal zinc deficiency, so this suggests that zinc is a vital nutrient for prostate health---at least as a preventative supplement.

The issue of "*high intensity chronic exercise...*" in this study is the only place where mention of a relationship between exercise and prostate cancer has been raised in the literature---it is not clear if physical exercise of all kinds are included in this link or if it pertains to (only)..."high intensity exercises that directly effect the prostate gland itself; like riding bicycles in high mileage or marathon races might do. But, someone should look at the relationship between cell damage in prostate cells of marathon bicycle racers to see if there is any possibility that that type of "high intensity chronic exercise" is, in fact, showing a higher incidence among those who participate and prostate cancer.

Since the remark appears only casually in the LPI research, the assumption can be made that there is little if any, evidence to show that routine exercising has any linkage to prostate cancer propagation. For the diagnosed man, certainly there is little reason to assume that cancer cells will spread more rapidly (or, for that matter, *less* rapidly) if routine exercise is continued. There are no studies yet that have examined this linkage sufficiently to make a prediction, one way or the other, so if part of your exercise routine is riding bicycles, you should feel safe in continuing to do so.

OTHER VITAMIN STUDIES

Most people have heard about the value of vitamin C and vitamin D, and vegetable-based enzymes in the liver that metabolize, detoxify, and help excrete carcinogens. Linus Pauling pioneered the use of vitamin C for treating all types of ills, including cancer in various parts of the body. In early work that Pauling and Ewan Cameron conducted, terminal cancer patients were treated with high dose intravenous and oral vitamin C where they found that many patients derived benefit from vitamin C, but those results were scattered: some patients benefited from an increased sense of well-being, others prolonged survival, and a few actually found that cancer went into regression, and a hand full went into remission. But, those kinds of results can be found in cancer patients who haven't routinely taken vitamin C, so the study had mixed results.

The Mayo Clinic released a large Vitamin C study in 2009 that said, essentially, that they could find little if any, benefit for vitamin C administered orally, even though there may be some 'halo' effect for some patients, in just making them have a 'sense of feeling better' and, in that sense, did not recommend against taking vitamin C supplements as part of a daily routine.

But, a more recent study by Mark Levine at the National Institutes of Health has elucidated how very high concentrations of vitamin C attained only by intravenous administration generates hydrogen peroxide around cancer cells that then kills them. The LPI researchers viewed this information as a mechanistic explanation for what vitamin C actually propagates at the cellular level and concluded that this knowledge will lead to better-designed clinical trials using intravenous vitamin C.

In other studies by J.D. Clarke and R.H. Dashwood, in the Emily Ho laboratory, studies are being conducted to see what happens to cancer cells if consumption of cruciferous vegetables, like broccoli, are controlled. Researchers know that stimulating myrosinase enzymes in the conciferous (broccoli) plant and gut microbes converts the parent compounds into sulforaphane. These compounds, in turn induce enzymes in the liver that metabolize, detoxify, and help excrete carcinogens much like a 'natural chemotherapy' that causes apoptosis (programmed cell death) ---which selective kills cancer cells.

So, this work is adding to the body of literature that supports what your mother has been telling you all these years: eat your vegetables! Unfortunately, the studies are not directed to specific organs (like the prostate gland) and are not yet large enough to draw conclusions about the efficacy of consumption of copious amounts of broccoli to effect killing off cancer cells.

Selenium is another essential mineral that humans get from their food intake. Unlike vitamin C and D, selenium is one of those that seems to have a delicate balance in the body: too much is bad, not enough is bad but no one seems to agree on exact levels for every person. Dashwood, et al is studying human colon cancer cells in selenium supplementation trials at the LPI lab but the results have been mixed. In this mechanistic study, two organic forms of selenium and their metabolites are being studied for their ability to inhibit histone deacetylase in human colon cancer cells. The inhibition of those histone deacetylase resulted in cell-cycle arrest and cell death but while the parent compounds did not appreciably effect histone deacetylase activity, the metabolites were inhibited in a dose-dependent manner that resulted in cell death. So, on the basis of this limited study, no recommendations about using selenium as either a prevention supplement or as a treatment supplement, can yet be offered.

One of the most trusted and authoritative sources of scientific studies on cancer and benefits from use of supplements is the Linus Pauling Institute at Oregon State University's Department of Biomedical Sciences. Assistant Senior Research Professor Debbie J. Mustacich, PhD., in the Institute's Department of Biomedical Sciences has studied the use of cisplatin in the treatment of a variety of solid tumors, including lung, ovarian and prostate cancer. In particular, she has found that cisplatin-based chemotherapy has been shown to significantly increase overall survival rates when used as adjuvant treatment in 'non-small-cell lung cancer (NSCLC) but also, in clinical trials has been demonstrated to increase response and median survival in hormone refractory prostate cancer (HRPC) patients treated with therapies that include platinum compounds (like the platinum-containing compound, cisplatin).

SUPPLEMENTATION STUDIES MIXED

Anecdotal evidence and single-case examples of vitamin supplements being effective in preventing or treating cancer appear throughout the literature. Today, the internet is rife with numerous stories of both real and made-up cancer remission caused by or effectively stemmed by, mega doses of various vitamins and/or herbals of all types and descriptions. One thing that is clear: the health human body requires varying levels of all essential vitamins and minerals, some of which should be supplemented and some that require no artificial supplementation if adequate exercise and sunshine are maintained.

The use of supplements as a cancer prevention tool or, for the cancer patient, as a dosing method like *natural chemotherapy* is being supported in the literature by study results that are just beginning to come from good scientifically designed studies. It is still unclear if supplementation is a silver bullet for treating cancer, but it is beginning to draw the attention of the mainstream medical community and clinical researchers so there is hope that the diagnosed person can look forward to more options for treatment in the coming years than are currently available.

FOODS AND SCIENCE: Got Milk?

"Cows milk is for cows." That's a quote you won't see in the American Dairy Association literature, but since we know so much about dairy products and their negative effects on the human body, milk is one of those 'foods' that is on the list of bad things you should not be consuming. And, its not just on a few lists; its on most nutritionist's, dietician's, naturopath's, and other professional's who see diet as one key to a healthy life. About the only medical professionals that think milk and milk products are OK for consumption are pediatricians who still refuse to look at the scientific evidence. The fact that a significant percentage of babies reject cow's milk (and must be fed lactose intolerance medicine or soy-based substitutes) should be enough evidence that, "cow's milk is (truly) for cows," and not humans.

Dairy products, especially cheese-based foods, which happen to be almost a 'staple' in our hectic fast-food life style (i.e. pizza and cheese-filled snack foods, cheese burgers and cheese-based Mexican food have become the best selling fast foods in the U.S.), make this diet staple a key player in the general population. And, by the way, according to Dr. Clapp (2000), studies have shown a high correlation between prostate cancer and dairy product consumption, so for our purposes, eliminating dairy products in men's diets should be considered a priority.

Lifestyle choices: Living A Healthy Life

In this section, we discuss some of the studies and literature that shows promise for 'prevention' of disease (primarily for cancer of the prostate). By illustrating where herbal remedies and Chinese medicines have been successful, we segue into cancer prevention through the use of these same techniques.

Alternative Medicine and Treatment Techniques

In recent times, the medical community has begun to embrace the use of here-to-fore unhearlded forms of treatment for all sorts of maladies. Notable among his peers, Dr. Andrew Weil at the University of Arizona Medical Center has been leading the way with incorporation of alternative medical techniques in his traditional practice. In addition, Dr. Dharma Singh Khalsa has also utilized 'meditation for medicine' techniques to help patients in the clinical setting.

ONCE AGAIN: Get More Than One Opinion

In keeping with our intent to be a 'primer' of information about male prostate disease(s) in general, and cancer of the prostate gland in particular, it should be painfully obvious that there is as much unknown as there is 'known' about prostate cancer. And, while that is obvious in the literature, the lay-public is mostly not aware that doctors (and medical community professionals, in general), are not accustomed to telling their patients that they don't have all the answers. But, it is true. The public has placed medical professionals on the elite pedestal for so long that its almost taken for granted that they are experts in every facet of medicine, even if they only profess to be specialists in one area of medical practice.

Interestingly, doctors (of all types) are allowed to "practice" their art, just as lawyers are allowed to "practice" law. Yet, we members of the lay-public (who become their patients and clients) are expected to fully trust their words as though they are infallible diagnosticians. Thus, if we allow ourselves to step back and take a deep breath whenever we are faced with diagnostics and prognostication from or about a serious medical condition, we allow ourselves to make choices such as seeking out second and third opinions, before we choose a therapy or treatment for the malady that has been diagnosed. So, men need to remember this before placing their blind faith in one doctor's opinion. Keep repeating: get another opinion! (And, another...and, another...etc.)

And, as noted earlier in this text, that is one of the most common problems with men when they are diagnosed with (prostate) cancer: they ask the doctor, *"what's my choice for treatment?"* and make the implicit assumption that this professional's opinion is infallible, since s/he has several years of medical school and years of experience to back it up. It is no different with trying to utilize any particular alternative medicine or alternative treatment: *there are no experts,* even among the 'doctors' and other 'medical professionals' that endorse a particular alternative treatment method.

DON'T ASK; DON'T TELL

Recently, the Newsletter from *Lets Talk Health* 2003, (www.letstalkhealth.com) featured an interview with several medical doctors on the general subject of prescription and alternative medications, and pharmaceutical industry costs. Dr. Jerry Avorn, a research physician at Harvard Medical School said it best about knowing what medications to prescribe:

> ***"If patients were aware of the limitations that all of us physicians have in terms of what we know and what we wish we knew and what we don't know, they would be more scared than they are at present. Always wait a year before prescribing a new drug, and if it is for a family member, wait five years! We really don't know as much as we would like to know about a drug until it's been around for awhile..."***

So, now you've heard it from the most prestigious of medical schools; prescription medications are a crap shoot and you need to be talking to your doctor AND your pharmacist to get all the right information.

Prevention and Alternative Medicine

Private herbal supply companies of all varieties have products purporting to be "the answer" to making your prostate healthy and/or preventing prostate cancer from occurring. Some purveyors provide charts and facts to back up their products. Since there is little scientific proof for such claims, its buyer beware. But, there are *'good sense'* precautions that can be taken and the use of the proper herbal products are among the best.

Researchers at the National Cancer Institute report that a diet with lots of vegetables from the allium food group, which includes garlic, shallots and onions, reduces the risk of prostate cancer by about half. The normal Chinese diet includes hearty servings of these vegetables. and previous studies have supported the general finding that eating vegetables is a good thing.

In this study which appeared in the Journal of the National Cancer Institute, 238 men with known prostate cancer and 471 men (thought to be) free of the disease, were interviewed. All the men in the study were residents of Shanghai, China and were asked how frequently they ate 122 food items.

The results showed that those who ate more than a third of an ounce a day from the allium food group were about 50 percent less likely to have prostate cancer than those who ate less of the foods. The conclusions still need to be replicated in further studies to be sure the results are statistically significant but the researchers believe, based on previous confirmatory research findings, that further research will bear out the fact that eating vegetables like scallions, onions, and garlic is prostate-cancer-preventative.

Other researchers at the Fred Hutchinson Cancer Research Center in Seattle confirmed that the results supports findings in some of their own studies: garlic and onions may be bad for your breath but they are good for your prostate! But, for the record, chlorophyll-coated garlic tablets are available that don't give you garlic breath!

ONE DOCTOR'S SOLUTION

It was mentioned before that there are numerous supplements that naturopathic physicians and even some mainstream doctors recommend for good prostate health. There are even some that have found considerable success with patients who have had their prostate removed but found, after years of PSA results 0.1 or less, that their PSA began to rise. One such case involved a man in the southeast who, eight years after having a radical prostatectomy, found his PSA values gradually rising (over a year's worth of PSA tests), from <1 to over 14, whereupon he consulted his surgeon. After x-rays and MRIs, and consultation with several doctors, it was decided that radiation of the groin area was required, even though no tumors were identified to be targeted. After 20+ radiation treatments, the man's bladder was so badly burned that the treatments were halted and the patient sought the help of the doctor at Lets Talk Health clinic via the radio program: www.letstalkhealth.com.

Dr. Donsbach, the *lets talk health* program's host and medical advisor, gave the man directions for taking an herbal supplement called prostasol which, he claims, is effective for stabilizing

PSA values in men who have had cancer treatment and for men who find their PSAs rising but have not yet been diagnosed with cancer.

In his radio program, Dr. Donsbach deals with all comers: whoever calls in with questions about any physical, or mental issue, receives advice for taking one or another of the many different herbal formulas that he sells---specific for any prostate issue is the herbal called prostasol---and without fail, is always prescribed for ANY prostate issue. This might include BPH issues, a urinary issue that appears to effect the prostate's seminal fluid pumping function, or the many ways PSA can be examined. In other words, it is not the intent of this book to endorse the product, prostasol, which Dr. Donsbach promotes but it IS important to give you information that might be useful for potentially effecting prostate cancer (or BPH symptoms) in a positive way.

Thus, you should know that prostasol, according to Dr. Donsbach, has been effective for reducing and stabilizing PSA values in men who have had surgery and in men who have not even been diagnosed. But, stabilizing PSA numbers is not necessarily the same thing as curing (or abating) cancer in the prostate. It is a well known fact that PSA is only an indicator that, statistically, has been shown to be right in 70% of men and wrong in 30% of men---but it is the best indicator screening test that medical science has been able to have confidence in---so, finding a drug or, in this case, a herbal supplement that stabilizes the PSA levels may be 90% effective in stopping the prostate specific antigen from being produced in the bloodstream, but not effective at all at killing cancer cells!

Dr. Donsbach has never claimed that prostasol does anything but stabilize PSA values over several months time, while getting PSA blood tests every three months, to see the trend in rising values stabilize around some constant number---he says, the number itself is of little importance---what is important is that it stabilizes and doesn't continue rising.

Thus, I put this information in this book to show you that there are doctors out there that you might consult, who have a good track record of giving you a product (a supplement) that gets outstanding results---but, those results must be evaluated for what they are and not for what you may want them to be. The point of this illustration is, always be sure you understand what it is that a given medicine or treatment, or supplement is supposed to be treating, BEFORE you pursue a given therapy. Some treatments may mask what is actually occurring and that could mean a delay in addressing the real problem.

This also illustrates what has been said and emphasized before: always seek more than one opinion before embarking on a treatment; there may be more harm in the 'treatment' than the cure it is supposed to effect.

LOOKING FOR SCIENCE: Ask the Scientists!

There are lots of reports in the papers these days about cancer and the relationship of foods we eat to both prevention and cures. Its not the purpose of this book to throw a lot of contradictory information out and confuse the issue so, in the interest of being as 'scientific' as possible, we've chosen to use the National Cancer Institute research and recommendations to summarize this controversial subject.

Here's the bottom line from NCI:

1.) Thirty percent or more cancers are linked to the foods we eat. Over the generations, the move from a diet high in plant-based foods to one significantly lower in plant foods may be one reason for higher rates of cancer.

2.) Vegetables, fruits, and whole grains contain essential vitamins and minerals as well as hundreds of phytochemicals that may protect against cancer and other chronic diseases such as heart disease.

3.) Over 200 studies worldwide clearly show that a plant-rich diet lowers the risk for numerous cancers. The key to this protection may be the way nutrients and phytochemicals in foods work together against cancer. NCI believes you can signifi cantly lower your risk of getting cancer by regularly eating certain foods and avoiding others.

4.) Reduced cancer risk can come from avoidance and reduction of consumption of fats, especially animal fats, red meat, grilled or overcooked meats, pickled and salt-cured meats, and those in which aflatoxins are present. In particular, evidence suggests that a diet high in fats may be linked to an increased risk of several cancers, prostate cancer included while red meats are linked to an increased risk of colon and prostate cancer.

5.) Reducing intake of (animal) fats and increasing fiber in the diet significantly reduces risk of cancer. Check the American Cancer Society and/or National Cancer Institute web sites for more information.

VITAMINS: Not a Substitute

We hear a lot these days about taking supplements – calcium, vitamin A, B, C, E, B-12, beta-carotene, antioxidants, free radical scavengers; etc. seem to be the subject of articles in the media every day. What is usually not apparent is, advice given about the value of taking these various and assorted 'supplements' almost lulls the reader into believing that, *'popping a few daily vitamins will substitute for not eating right!'*

Nothing could be further from the truth. Thus, for our purposes here, there are some basic truths we need to state: supplemental vitamins may be essential for most people because most of us do not eat properly and tend not to get the daily ration of what the experts think is essential. But (and it is a very BIG, *'BUT!'*), supplements are not a substitute for eating the proper diet, especially the proper foods that lower cancer risk (as noted before in this chapter).

Most nutritionists and, indeed, most physicians who know the value of foods in preventive medicine, agree that there are 13 essential nutrients which the body cannot make in adequate amounts for the body's daily needs, let alone in amounts that are considered *cancer risk preventative*.

In addition, there are others – perhaps as many as 17 or 18 – that are only stored in the body for a short time, before they 'wash' out so they need replenishment more often, and supplements can provide those.

HERBS AND HERBALS

There is a difference in vitamins and herbs, even though the mass media seems to lump the two into the same class of "supplemental health aids." The distinction may be subtle; many vitamins are actually made of herbal ingredients. However, for our purposes, it is important that men facing dietary decisions to combat prostate cancer, understand the distinction. Vitamins can be thought of as, classically, those things that the USDA says our bodies require. We see these in advertisements as "recommended Daily Dose" for Vitamin B, Vitamin C, Vitamin E; etc., etc.

Herbs may also be a "vitamin" or be an ingredient in a particular vitamin complex, but they may also be considered "food" that the body uses to enhance overall health or, health of particular organs. Just as Vitamin C is required for healthy bones and teeth, an herb like saw palmetto has been used both as a preventive and corrective for prostate problems. By building the thyroid to control the operation of glands, saw palmetto helps overcome such men's health problems as enlarged prostate, underdeveloped testicles, sterility and impotence.

BPH AND SUPPLEMENTS

According to Nature's Field Distributor's Newsletter (March/April 1999), saw palmetto has been shown in studies in Europe to be more effective for BPH sufferers than the drug (proscar) most often recommended to relieve this condition. (See also Potter's New Encyclopedia of Botanical Drugs and Preparations by R.C. Wrens; Essex, England; C.W. Daniel Company Limited, 1985).

Other BPH herbals include combinations of horsetail herb, black cohosh root, uva ursi leaves, licorice root, kelp plant, capsicum fruit, golden seal root, and ginger root. Other herbs that have been shown in studies to help overcome prostate problems include stinging nettle (which does not sting when its taken in dried form), and gotu kola (hydrocotyle asiatica) is another herbal preparation which can be used for enlarged prostate. Many prostate-specific herbal combinations are, in fact, available from stores and naturopathic clinics that specialize in glandular problem prevention and/or cancer treatment.

As was mentioned earlier in this chapter, one supplement that is recommended by one doctor may be useful for treating both BPH and cancer. That supplement is called Prostasol and may or may not be everything its advertising says, but it seems to be successful for some men, based on the manufacturer's claims.

An excellent source of information on herbs and supplements and their use for cancer treatment and cancer prevention is Miracle Cures written by Jean Carper and published by Harper-Collins in 1997. It is still in print and still referenced in medical clinics for prostate health advice. It has one whole chapter devoted to prostate health, with herbs and supplements and includes documentation of the studies which support the findings.

Of course, so-called case studies have been used in other papers and books about the "miracle cure of the month" but Carper's book provides documentation and reports on controlled studies to support most of her case studies. For example, she cites vitamin studies conducted at the

University of Virginia, and selenium studies at the University of Arizona, among others in showing the success of dietary changes in eradicating cancer.

In addition, there are studies conducted by Dr. Keith Block at the Cancer Institute in Chicago that have shown success in cancer treatment in a variety of patients for various herbals and supplements. The evidence is mounting: herbs and supplements are being used with conventional cancer therapies to combat cancer and decrease side effects of radiation treatments.

WATERMELON: Sweet Lycopene

Tomatoes get the headlines for their protective effect against prostate cancer, but *"ounce for ounce, watermelon contains 40% more of the active cancer-fighting compound lycopene than tomatoes,"* according to Dr. David Kiefer, a fellow in the University of Arizona's Program in Integrative Medicine. Kiefer is a researcher in the program headed by alternative medicine guru Andrew Weil, M.D., and says that their studies show that not only is lycopene crucial in overall prostate health. Kiefer suggests that "other studies are showing that it may block the plaque buildup in arteries that can lead to heart attack and it may offset some of the cellular damage and aging effects that lead to Alzheimer's, Parkinson's, and arthritis." (AARP, Sept/Oct 2003)

VITAMINS SHOWN IN STUDIES TO REDUCE PROSTATE CANCER ***RISK***

There have been several studies that have shown that certain vitamins reduce the risk of getting cancer and reports from NCI, ACS, and some like the London Hospital research, which have shown promise for prostate cancer specifically. The vitamin which has shown the most promise as a preventative, and for which there seems to be the most scientific evidence, is Vitamin E. In studies cited by Richard Harkness, Steven Bratman and David Kroll in *The Natural Pharmacist* (also available on www.TNP.com on the internet), a 1998 study in Finland of more than 36,000 adults found that a diet low in vitamin E increased overall cancer risk by 50%!

They also cited a study of 11,178 elderly individuals who reported taking vitamin E had an overall 59% reduction in cancer deaths. Even after adjusting the data for alcohol use, smoking history, aspirin use and other medical conditions, the results were the same. The researchers concluded that vitamin E supplements could also help prevent death from heart disease in this same study.

In a study of 29,000 male smokers in Finland who took supplements of either 50 mg of vitamin E, 20 mg of betacarotene, both or a placebo daily for 5 to 8 years, there was a 32% lower incidence of prostate cancer and a 41% fewer prostate cancer deaths. They also reported, surprisingly, that the positive results came soon after the start of supplementation and have concluded that the vitamin E might block the progression of the slow-growing prostate cancer cells (although this conclusion is not supported by the study itself).

They have also speculated that, because this study was aimed at looking at smokers and the impact of vitamin E on lung cancer, it is reasonable to think that vitamin E might work even better on non-smokers. Studies are underway currently, to replicate the results.

The fact is, even if all those studies are accurate, they don't give the cancer victim who has cancer any information about what the effect of those vitamins and herbals might have on treating cancer that is already diagnosed. But, for the BPH sufferer or the man who wants to do everything he can to prevent the risk of getting prostate cancer, these studies offer a life-style menu of dietary options that just might reduce the odds that someday you won't have to hear those terrible words from your physician.

SUMMARIZING SCIENCE

Studies are accumulating from reputable institutions that are showing that what we eat may have a major role to play in both, cancer prevention and cancer cure. Specific studies have been cited by the National Cancer Institute (NCI) and the American Cancer Institute (ACI) and, as well, at private research centers in the U.S. and Europe which are showing that the evidence supporting the role of food and nutrients (i.e. supplements) for cancer prevention is growing.

New research at traditional medical institutions where non-traditional medicine is playing a significant role, is breaking ground every day. Andrew Weil at the University of Arizona Medical Center, prostate cancer research at Cedars Sinai in Los Angeles supported by the Michael Milken Foundation, NCI-funded prostate research at the Cleveland Institute and the J. Hayden Fry Center for Prostate Cancer Research at the University of Iowa (U of I) are just a few of the newest efforts to find preventative techniques and treatments for prostate cancer.

Recently, the National Institutes of Health awarded the U of Iowa $2.5 million to study whether phytotherapy is effective in treating the enlarged prostate (i.e. BPH). There are actually 10 institutions nationwide participating in the Complimentary and Alternative Medicines for Urology Symptoms study so we are hopeful that one of the study spin-offs will show the validity of using phytotherapy (i.e. the use of plant extracts) for treating prostate cancer, too.

With the national effort toward *curing* cancers of all types, and the encouraging new research efforts utilizing diet and supplement research for prostate cancer *prevention*, we can be optimistic that prostate cancer can one day be eradicated. Until that time comes, diet and nutrition certainly needs to be a part of every man's risk reduction plan because, if it is not a part of the solution, diet is most certainly a part of the problem.

REALITY: DRUGS ARE BIG BUSINESS

You've seen the statistics and every day in TV news and in the newspapers, we are bombarded with advertising by pharmaceutical companies about specific drugs they are claiming you can not live without. *"Ask your doctor..."* they all say, implying that your doctor is going to endorse their prescription medication for you. How much more confidence could you have that those medical professionals once again have your best interests at heart? Little wonder that its difficult to get good research (data) on alternative medicines when main stream drug companies exert such control over funding.

But, realize that consumers spent $90 Billion more on prescription drugs in 2001 than they did five years before, in 1996! Sure, you say, but drug companies need to get their research investment back for the millions they spent developing those great drugs. But, that's before you realize that the drug industry spent $15 Billion in 2001 in advertising to get you to ask for particular drugs and to get doctors to prescribe them! Does all this paint a picture of collusion between the medical practicioners and drug companies, with *you* playing the role of guinea pig in the middle? And, who's paying for it? You guessed it! We guinea pigs!

Dr. Drummond Rennie is one of the editors at the Journal of the American Medical Association (JAMA) who's not afraid to state the obvious: He says researchers who are critical of the establishment get attacked all the time. *"I believe."* he's quoted on www.letstalkhealth.com (July, 2003) as saying, that *"...drug companies are intent on keeping the consumer on drugs, for the simple requirement of profit."*

And that's from the JAMA, one of the most quoted and prestigious of medical journals of research in the world. Is it any wonder that *herbal* therapies get such bad press?

A Case History That You Should Know About

While putting the finishing touches on this *Second Edition*, I found an advertisement for a small book called ***CANCER*** by Tommy Johnson Sr.

This small book is written from the heart and, therefore, is not about the 'scientific' findings that support a specific treatment or drug but it explores the 'process' that a positive diagnosis causes a man to go through while, at the same time, provides detailed information on various prescriptive medications and alternative drugs and therapies that may offer treatment alternatives that have not been explored elsewhere in Prostate Cancer 2.0..

Tommy's cancer was not in his Prostate; he was diagnosed with Stage 4 Colon Cancer and given a short-term survival prognosis that sent him into a deep depression. The fact that he chose to detail his journey through conventional treatment and into alternative treatment therapies and that his successful, step by step decision-making has rewarded him with 10+ years of cancer in remission means that this book should be a part of any cancer library resources. So it is highly recommended and some of his journey highlights are provided here because his views are consistent with the message of Prostate Cancer 2.0: seek second and third opinions and thoroughly do your research to find the best cancer treatment therapies for your own situation.

The essential ingredients in Tommy's book (and journey) that make it useful here are in the various alternative therapies that he discovered which, according to Tommy, saved his life and has allowed him to live a very enjoyable and pain-free existence in the 10 years following his bleak diagnosis.

Tommy (and other cancer victims) was advised that the (then) new drug that might have an effect on his longevity was, Laetrile, a commercial name for amygdalin that has actually been banned by the FDA from being used on humans but is still approved for veterinary use on animals. Thus, while it can not be prescribed by physicians, it is still 'available' for your animals if you want to experiment.

It is also readily available from Mexico and Tommy's provided his sources in his book in case that is something you want to pursue. As noted, his cancer was not in his Prostate so none of his research has been directed at use of various alternative therapies for Prostate Cancer. The fact is, however, that his journey process is worth looking at, even if the end result is not taking amygdalin (or some have labeled it Vitamin B-17).

It is available through a number of web sites but heed Tommy's warning: not ALL websites are honest and therefore, you need to do your homework before taking some unknown product that may do you more harm than good. Here is a website that Tommy recommends: http://www.cytopharma.com/amygdalin.htm

Another herbal 'ingredient' that is crucial also contains some of the same amygdalin as the laetrile capsules and comes from Apricot Seed kernels. Although the FDA has not yet banned the sale and use of apricot seed kernels, so they are available from health food stores and websites.

Tommy's successful struggle to find a way to treat his colon cancer is a story that should give every Prostate Cancer victim hope that, just because some therapies haven't been documented in the literature for one kind of cancer, doesn't mean those same therapies might not work when applied to another. Tommy's use of laetril, along with a few other herbal treatment and exercise regimes, just might be a silver bullet for case-specific situations where all the other therapies have failed.

So, while the research conducted in compiling the studies and therapies for this Second Edition didn't reveal any where that laetrile had been used to successfully treat Prostate Cancer, there were no cases where laetrile was specifically noted in treatment schemes that resulted in either successful or not successful treatment of PC. Therefore, it is offered here as one man's hope that the search for successful treatment therapies will never end: buy Tommy's book and send him continued good wishes for good health.

RUNNING FROM CANCER: Walking May Be As Good

In the May, 2003 edition of Energy Times (pp 70), studies by the UCLA Jonsson Cancer Center and Department of Physiological Science have found that a strict walking regimen, along with a high-fiber, low fat diet, can slow the growth of prostate cancer cells by up to 30%. According to William Aronson, the senior study author, the study, strongly suggests that a low-fat diet and exercise regimen appears to favorably affect the levels of hormones or growth factors that influence prostate cancer growth" (Journal of Urology 2001; 166(3): 1185-9).

The article points out also that in Boston, an investigation that followed almost 4,000 women for 15 years found that those who had been athletes in their college days suffered 17% less breast cancer than women who had not engaged in college sports. Co-author of the study, Grace Wyshak from the Harvard School of Public Health "looked at more than 20 studies, and the weight of evidence suggests that regular physical activity does offer some protection against (breast) cancer." (British Journal of Cancer, 2000; 82(3): 726-30)

In these times when everyone is so busy with leisure-time activities, the National Center for Health Statistics points out that more than 30% of all men and 40% of all women report not exercising at all. The evidence from UCLA and Boston's Harvard Medical School would seem to spur both men and women in their 30's, 40's, 50's, and 60's to reprioritize their leisure-time activities. Its pretty clear that successful preventative measures are related to a combination of diet and exercise. Its only a matter of mind over matter: in light of all the evidence that's mounting, it is clear that we must *prevent* cancer or suffer the consequences!

NATIONAL CANCER INSTITUTE: Focus on Red Meat

As noted before, some of the studies that have been conducted by the National Cancer Institute have been designed to study the effects of a person's diet on risk of cancer. Recently, NCI studies show that people who ate the most red meat, averaging at least 3 ounces daily of especially well-done or fried red meats, had twice the risk of colon cancer compared with those who ate less than half an ounce daily.

A study that NCI sponsored at the VA Medical Center in Portland, Oregon, also indicated that breast cancer risk doubled in postmenopausal women who ate 3 ounces or more of red meat a day compared with women who consumed one ounce or less daily. This study tended to confirm the results of a Vanderbilt University study that concluded that women who ate the most deep-fried, well-done, meat had nearly twice the probability of developing breast cancer as those who ate the least.

In another study conducted at the University of Minnesota, eating broiled red meat did not increase the risk of pancreatic cancer but the odds doubled in people who ate the most grilled or barbecued red meat.

All these studies seem to say that meaty diets, particularly red meat diets like the Atkins High protein diet, increase the risk of cancer (but its not something you read in the Atkins Diet Books). So, if you are a "meat and potatoes" man, what should you do?

MEAT, HEAT, AND NITROSAMINES: What Science Is Saying

According to Jean Carper (jeancarper.com) who writes and researches literature in the sciences, there are ways to sidestep cancer and (still) pack in the protein. Here's some of Carper's advise from *Eat Smart*, USA Weekend Magazine (Jul 4-6, 2003)

1. Eat fish or poultry (and little or NO red meat):

   In particular, Carper says that women who ate fish three or more times weekly had a 30% lower breast cancer risk than women who ate fish once a week in the VA study in Oregon. In another study (not identified by Carper), eating chicken baked, broiled or barbecued did not raise colon cancer risk while pan-frying chicken boosted odds 50%.

2. Eat meat rare or medium rare and cook it slowly:

   At high heats (as in frying), proteins form heterocyclic amines or HCA's, which are potent carcinogens. Thus, reduced heat creates fewer HCA's with broiling producing fewer carcinogens than grilling. In the University of Minnesota study, consistently eating hamburger, beef steak and bacon very well done, instead of rare or medium, increased women's breast cancer risk almost five times.

3. Eat turkey or soy burgers but not hamburgers:

   The goal is to cut down on the formation of carcinogens which are formed in the cooking process, particularly at high heat. If you mix antioxidants like soy protein, mashed blueberries or cherries, tea, garlic or onions into beef burger meat before cooking, Carper says you can cut the formation of carcinogens by 60% to 90% and that reduces your risk of cancer.

4. Pre-cook meat you are going to grill:

   Since pre-cooking meat before its grilled cuts down on the formation of those cancer-causing HCA's, pop your meat into a microwave and pre-cook it before you grill it.

5. Use *"watery"* sauces instead of heavy past-sauces before grilling:

   Carper notes that some research has shown that thick tomato barbecue sauce may foster carcinogen formation (Carper noted no research citation).

6. Avoid nitrite-cured meats:

   Even (the late) Dr. Atkins recommended using nitrite-free bacon from health-food stores. Most cured cold cuts, hot dogs, bacon, and ham also contain nitrites that can spur formation of nitrosamines that are known carcinogens so, Carper notes, whenever possible, look for nitrite-free meats.

CAUTIONARY NOTES

We conclude this section on a cautionary note. The literature today on diets runs the gamut from one extreme to another. The information recently that testosterone hormone therapy (for men) is beginning to be as popular with men as hormone replacement therapy (for women) is, or was, in women. But, recently, there have been side effects reported in men who used testosterone (hormone) therapy to increase their libido; there are varying opinions about unintended consequences. Doctors either like hormone replacement therapy for menopausal women or they don't like it and there seems to be much debate with studies that support both views.

With men, testosterone (hormones), or the diminished production of them, are thought to be the cause for everything from loss of sex drive to loss of body hair. Over the past few years, testosterone prescriptions have become increasingly popular with doctors. In 2002, almost 600,000 men age 45 and older used some form of prescription testosterone to raise the level of the sex hormone in their bodies, and the number is rising every year. By 2010, that number nearly doubled and more than a million men are using some kinds of prescription hormone on a daily basis! And, that doesn't include the thousands of men (and women) who are buying over-the-counter sex hormones.

Dr. Stanley Slater, is a top scientist/researcher at the National Institute on Aging (NIA) and Deputy Associate Director of NIA's geriatrics and clinical gerontology program who has probably studied testosterone's effects on men longer than almost anyone else. He notes (in Your Health, AARP Bulletin/July-August 2003, pp 16-18), that there are safety issues to be addressed. In particular, "we know that testosterone feeds the growth of tumors in men who have metastatic prostate cancer." Thus, he cautions, "that most older men harbor inactive and harmless "'nests"' of prostate cancer cells and by giving extra testosterone to these men (to help their libido), "we don't know if we're awakening a sleeping monster."

On the other hand, Dr. Slater doesn't specialize in prostate cancer treatment or prescribe therapies for victims of prostate cancer, so no studies have been conducted that link the use of hormone therapy with increasing levels of tumor growth (either inside or outside the prostate capsule). What we do know is, a hormone shot is administered almost immediately to the prostate cancer patient whose biopsy and body scans both indicate that the cells have migrated outside the prostate. It is still the most effective and quickest method of stopping cell growth. For that patient, the concern about the hormone's effect on increasing cell growth may be moot; if the hormone shot stops the cancer, there is no need for further study!

In early 2004, however, NIH canceled a major large-scale trial after questions were raised about its design and the director of NCI opposed it because of prostate cancer worries. It seems that scientists cannot agree on what testosterone is good for, since administering a hormone shot effectively stops cancer cells dead in their tracks. On the other hand, thousands of men are using testosterone in all different types of applications that result in renewed vigor which makes men feel young again. For cancer victims, however, there are no scientific answers and hormone shots remain the only high percentage method of stopping prostate cancer cells; stay tuned for further information from the scientists who continue to look for cures.

FROM THE MILKEN FOUNDATION RESEARCH

In the First Edition of this book, it was noted that the Milken Family Foundation has provided funding for prostate cancer research since the mid-1980's, totaling more than $100 Million. Among its funded research projects, they have supported numerous nutrition studies and have amassed a very large data base of nutritional information. In addition to their own studies, available at their web site at www.milkenfoundation.com, they also publish numerous web sites where information can be found on general diets and nutrition.

For instance, in mid-2003, the site listed the following:

Web Site URL	Description of Information Available
www.miavita.com	This is a client-based site that provides healthy living information and nutrition ideas for employees and clients of Miavita Corporation. The info is provided free simply by going to their web site address.
www.navigator.tufts.edu	This site is maintained by nutritionists at Tufts University that provides numerous other nutrition web sites that give clear and concise information on diet and nutrition.
www.soyfoods.com	Maintained by the Indiana Soy Bean Board offers a complete directory of manufacturers of soy products like tofu and tempeh.
www.envirolinks.org.orgs.vegweb	Online guide to vegetarianism provides more than 2000 recipes, weekly meal planners, and gardening information.
www.eatright.org/index	This is the website for the world's largest organization of dieticians with a directory of members.

Also available on the Milken Foundation site are the two cookbooks that Michael Milken (compiled by Beth Ginsberg) called **The Taste For Living World Cookbooks**, specifically for helping to fight prostate cancer. Additionally, a PDF-formatted report is available that compiles prostate-specific related nutritional information that may be helpful to sufferers with enlarged prostates as well as cancer.

All the work done by the CaP Cure research sponsored by the Milken Foundation is clinic-tested and has been a tremendous help in the battle against prostate cancer so, men facing prostate treatment decisions must take advantage of the tremendous resources the Milken Foundation provides.

THE BEST OF THE BEST

Besides the work funded by the Milken Foundation, or should we say *"including"* the Milken Foundation efforts through CaP CURE, there are studies being conducted in several traditional medical settings using herbs and alternative therapies for prostate cancer. Among the top research clinics that are focused on controlled studies that use herbs in the treatment of prostate cancer is one that stands out: The Jonsson Cancer Center at the University of California-Los Angeles (UCLA).

The Jonsson Cancer Center, (available on the Web at www.cancer.mednet.ucla.edu), was named by U.S. News and World Report as one of the top ten cancer centers in America (Jul 21, '03 USNews.com). The rankings are charted by 150 leading physicians practicing oncology through out more than 50 medical cancer centers in the U.S. The Jonsson Center was rated the best in California among five others that were ranked in the top 50 in the survey.

The top ten centers nationally are the M.D. Anderson Cancer Center, Houston, TX (1); Memorial Sloan-Kettering Center, New York, (2); Johns Hopkins Hospitals, Baltimore, MD, (3); Dana-Farber Cancer Institute, Boston, MA, (4); Mayo Clinic, Rochester, MN, (5); University of Chicago, Chicago, IL, (6); Duke University Medical Center, Durham, NC, (7); UCLA Jonsson Cancer, Los Angeles, CA, (8); University of Michigan Medical Center, Ann Arbor, MI, (9); and Vanderbilt University Medical Center, Nashville, TN, (10).

It should be noted that, while all the cancer centers in the rankings treat prostate cancer, the Jonsson Center has a special program aimed at conducting research specifically utilizing alternative therapies and, most importantly, herbal formulations for prostate cancer. Their research is mainstream medical studies using "good scientific principles" to achieve peer-reviewed and credible scientific results. On their website, they encourage interested patients to apply and become part of clinical studies and their overall approach is aimed at learning how to reduce and/or prevent mortality from prostate cancer.

It should also be noted that the Jonsson website has links to a variety of medical journals and sources of cancer information. The herbal cancer study, either accessed through the Jonsson Center website or directly on the internet can be found at www.canceralternatives.mednet.ucla.edu and includes information on what herbs are being studied. The good news is, the mainstream medical community is beginning to integrate herbal therapies into treatment and prevention of cancer of all kinds and, it appears that the UCLA Jonsson Cancer Center is leading the effort.

Recent news from the Jonsson Cancer Center includes an announcement that, for the second year in a row, the doctors and prostate cancer researchers have received the largest grant of any other single institution nationwide. A grant totaling $1 Million was awarded by CaP CURE, the Michael Milken Foundation that is profiled elsewhere in this text. Dr. Charles Sawyers, head of the Prostate Cancer Center at the Jonsson Center, noted that:

> **"(...the combined research at the Center)** ***has been providing new insights into molecular disease mechanisms (represented in prostate cancer) and targeted organs such as breast cancer, leukemia, and lymphoma and its easy to envision how these same strategies might be brought to bear on prostate cancer*** **(with the new monies provided by CaP Cure added to existing funding.)"**

The herbal studies program, announced in January, 2003, was funded with $1.1 Million and is being carried out at the Sue Stiles Program in Integrative Oncology and, according to a news release ((www.nbc4tv.health), will focus on:

> ***"...an untapped goldmine of plant life and natural compounds that haven't been tested as potential cancer fighters....such things as components of shark liver oil, soy and yerba santa, a plant historically used by Native Americans for healing.***

In a comment by the Director of Integrative Oncology at the Jonsson Center, Dr. Richard Pietras noted that,

> ***" These plants and compounds could one day replace more toxic and debilitating chemotherapies now in use...I hope that we will one day be able to treat cancer patients with less harmful and more targeted therapies to fight their tumors and relieve their symptoms."***

Dr. Pietras also noted that:

> ***"... of the 92 drugs approved for cancer treatment from 1983 to 1994, 62 were derived from natural sources and...more than 50 Million compounds have never been screened for tumor-fighting properties (in controlled studies)."***

It is encouraging that the mainstream medical community is recognizing the importance of herbs and supplements as valid medical prescription alternatives.

"IF YOU HAVE BEEN DIAGNOSED WITH CANCER (ANY CANCER... NOT *ONLY* PROSTATE CANCER), YOU ABSOLUTELY *MUST* SEEK MORE THAN ONE MEDICAL OPINION ABOUT YOUR TREATMENT OPTIONS! AND, YOU ABSOLUTELY *MUST* SEEK OPINIONS FROM DIFFERENT TREATMENT SPECIALISTS: SURGERY, RADIATION, CRYOGENICS, ROBOTICS SURGERY; ETC."

CHAPTER SEVEN

Exciting New Therapies For Prostate Cancer

...In this chapter, you will learn about....

FUTURE TREATMENTS: Cryogenics, Vaccines, Robot-Assisted RP....

PHOTODYNAMIC THERAPY

Turn Up The Heat

SNAKE OIL: BEWARE!

GOOD NEWS FOR PROSTATECTAMIES (And Other Treatments, too!)

Upside verses Downside: You Decide

INTRODUCTION

Researchers at University College London Hospital in England have been treating many types of cancer, including prostate cancer, with a method they have labeled ***'photodynamic therapy'*** (PDT). At the London hospital, they used the therapy on 14 men whose prostate cancer had come back after being treated with radiation. First, the patients got an intravenous injection of the photosensitive drug, then they waited three days for the drug to migrate into the tumor(s). At that point, the doctors shined (laser) light on the tumors to activate the photosensitive drug, which destroys the tumors.

It is still in the development stages but researchers believe PDT will have few complications or side-effects, once the therapy is perfected. So, it appears this therapy not only has great promise for the patient who has previously been treated for cancer of the prostate but also as a possible treatment for newly discovered prostate cancer which is contained within the capsule.

Many more trials and more research remains to be done, but this is probably one of the highest probability therapies with the greatest promise for prostate cancer treatment that is being studied at the present time.

TURN UP THE HEAT

There is an interesting internet web site that features a Naturopathic Physician answering questions about alternative medicine and treatments for all kinds of maladies, including cancer. In a recent issue of www.letstalkhealth.com (Volume 5, Number 3 Newsletter) editor Kurt W. Donsbach discussed the use of an old treatment called Delwa-Star H & P thermo-therapy for treating hemorrhoids. Dr. Donsbach noted also that, recently, he had seen dramatic results when the 'device' was used for prostatic hypertrophy. The thermotherapy is based on the concept that an increase in temperature of the tissue produces an irrigation of blood to the area concerned and relaxes the musculature around it, allowing an even greater flow. Dr. Donsbach notes that when the thermotheraputic probe was applied for consecutive periods of time, there was an observed reduction in the prostate (size) and "actually reverses itself thereby relieving symptoms (of BPH)…" and side effects.

Donsbach indicated that *"the concept is proven now for both hemorrhoids and prostatic conditions,"* although he does not cite any specific studies supporting his thesis. It is unclear whether any studies have been done on the use of thermotheraputic probes for prostate cancer but, in most men over the age of 70, cancer is almost always preceded by lengthy problems with BPH. Thus, it is possible that shrinking the gland by thermotheraputic applications may slow or even eliminate the onset of cancer in the gland. Again, no studies are cited and none have been found in the literature although several cancer clinics indicated they are experimenting with thermo-treatment applications for prostate cancer.

SNAKE OIL: BEWARE!

In medicine, cures for every malady known to man (and woman) have been touted for centuries throughout history by charlatans of every kind. Most "remedies" turned out to be shams to make the morbidity of the general public a cash cow for the purveyors. Today, with the tremendous growth of the World Wide Web (Internet) just in this new millennium, literally thousands of web sites are touting cancer cures that rival all the snake oil salesmen that ever plied their trade.

Recently, the AARP surfed the Internet to see what's being "sold" as sure-fire cancer cures and they were amazed to learn that, *"what's eluded the world's leading medical researchers around the globe is already available, and in more than one "clinical" setting: a cure for cancer!"* (AARP Journal, January 2003).

There are "cures" that are available from both women and men who've found *the answer* (to various cancer-types, including prostate cancer), for the low, low price of $18.95 and there are cures that use everything from powdered shark cartilage to hydrazine sulfate that are "guaranteed" to eradicate cancer, almost overnight! Some cancer products and therapy sites sell videos that promise, much like the circus barkers, that cancer will virtually "leap right out of the body," right before your very eyes!

Just in case you are tempted to spend your money, you probably should check with other authorities, like the FTC, before you send in a check. The Bulletin also notes that a good place to learn about cancer quackery is right on the internet, available at www.quackwatch.org.

All this is not to say there isn't good information or, perhaps, even remedies for prostate cancer that have no clinical trials or history yet which are being looked at by very good research clinics. There are many great hospitals and clinics who have web sites, some that have been referenced in this book, so the message is: be cautious when conducting your research on the Internet. It's a whole new world of possibilities and you deserve not to be scammed.

In the final analysis, if you think you have been diagnosed with prostate cancer, use any and all means of getting good information about your options. And good health and a long life is our wish for you!

AFTER A PROSTATECTOMY: WHAT IF??

Let's just think about the unthinkable: what if a prostatectomy has been performed and has resulted in the dreaded "erectile dysfunction" (ED). What's the prognosis for a cure?

Recently, there have been studies using Viagra (sildenafil) for prostate cancer patients, after treatment. Reuters Health (New York, April, 2003) studied men for nine months after having their prostates removed and found some interesting results. The study was conducted by Dr. Harin Padma-Nathan of the University of Southern California in LA where they asked 23 and 28 men to take 50 milligrams and 100 milligrams of Viagra, respectively, every night for nine months, starting four weeks after the radical prostatectomy. Another 25 men took a placebo during the same time period. None of the men knew whether they were taking Viagra or a placebo and all of the men had normal erectile function before surgery.

Padma-Nathan discovered that 27 % of men who had received Viagra, regardless of dose (some were given 100 mls and some were given 50 mls), had regained full erectile functioning, equal to what they reported before undergoing surgery while only 4% of the men given the placebo recovered erectile function.

No serious side effects were reported by any of the Viagra group and Padma-Nathan concluded that, "doing nothing is not good. Intervention (i.e. using Viagra) certainly made it a whole lot better."

Given that the men in the study were in their mid-50's, it means there is hope for resumption of a normal sex life after prostate surgery, although there is an expense associated with Viagra. On the other hand, Padma-Nathan noted that animal studies have shown that the drug may actually be restoring or reattaching nerves that are damaged in the surgery, thereby giving hope that the medication may actually "fix" the problem and erectile function might return without intervention later on. Of course, its too soon to tell if that's possible, but there's hope.

The good news is, use of sildenfil for prostate cancer treated with other means, like brachytherapy or E Beam, can provide even stronger erections, especially in the early months following treatment. And it is yet another opportunity to show that the medical community is moving forward in prostate cancer *recovery* research even as new cancer elimination treatments are being found.

PARTING SHOTS

It has been said in other parts of this Prostate Cancer 2.0 that, because men are the way they are, almost anything of a medical nature that affects areas *"below the belt"* and above the knees, is ginger territory; they don't want to talk about it or deal with it. Women, on the other hand, because of their very biological differences, seem to be more at ease in dealing with problems in those areas of their bodies.

Men also are used to hearing all the jokes and, over the years of growing into a fully functional sexual animal, have seen and heard all the penis jokes and urban legends. Believe it or not, many men also still believe in the adage that "bigger is better" when it comes to penis size, although women (at least when asked if that would be their personal belief), would be mostly reluctant to endorse such statements.

The literature is vague on this as it relates to prostate cancer treatment(s) but in discussions with both doctors who perform radical prostatectamies and with men who have had that surgery, it is fairly common knowledge that erections (post-operative) result in shorter penis length by one to two inches, on average (based on those self-descriptions). And that is based upon a very 'small' survey---most men who were interviewed for this book, were hesitant to discuss their sex life (post-prostatectemy or otherwise)----and several had not experienced an erection so had no idea whether or not the length of their penis has been effected, one way or the other.

For those few who did discuss this sensitive subject, who actually had experienced erections after having surgery, every one of them agreed that their penis 'length' had been reduced as well as rigidity being less---several had indicated that using Viagra or Calias became a necessary part of foreplay---but partner satisfaction seemed to vary from person to person, and partner to partner.

For brachytherapy, there appears to also be a reduction in length but perhaps less than one and a half inches in length, although the rigidity of the erection also seems to be diminished somewhat from before the implanted seeds procedure was performed. But, the small sample of couples interviewed said, basically, they were satisfied that their 'performance' in the boudoir was as good as before brachytherapy with most men (and their partners), saying they've had no complaints.

The literature is silent on both these issues but the anecdotal evidence is fairly consistent. So, should that impact a man's decision (or a couple) on which treatment to choose? Of course not! But, it is an issue you won't find discussed anywhere else, at least not in popular literature dealing with prostate cancer.

Flaccid State May Be Worse Than Any!

Now here is where I need to make you aware of a potential problem, no matter which treatment you use for your PC: urologists will not agree with me on this because they "have no data…" to prove cause and effect but, the penis in the flaccid state (i.e. 'soft' or not erect), will tend to "shrink" over time and just being able to 'extend' the penis for urination can sometimes be a problem for the man who has had any PC treatment procedure (emphasis on ANY). My interviews with men about the general subject of 'effects' on the 'length of the penis' after treatment, whether radical surgery, robotic surgery, E-Beam, Brachytherapy or Cryogenic, revealed the following general concensus:

The length of the penis in the sexually aroused position generally was 1 ½" to 2" less with a radical (surgery), about ½" to 1" less for Brachytherapy patients and E-Beam, and about the same for other treatments like cryogenics. One would think this would be a concern to most men (and their partners) but, it turns out that the men interviewed for this Edition 2.0 who had one or another of the PC treatments actually said their 'sexual' experience post-PC-treatment was about what they'd been expecting, with surgery patients having the least success and those who had brachytherapy having the most (or least problems) sexual satisfaction, post-treatment. What was unexpected, though, was the results of asking: what problems or issues have you had, post-treatment, with your penis (length, urination, use)? Here is a general synopsis of their answers:

> The length of the penis in the 'normal' (flaccid) state is very difficult to measure (of course) but to a man---every man interviewed for this book, admittedly a small sample of post-treatment men numbering between 12 and 18 men ranging in age from 58 to 75---said there was a tendency for their penis to 'retreat' inside the pubic cavity which, for some (7 of 12 asked this question), made it very difficult to 'pull' the penis out far enough to be able to urinate while in a standing position. Some men experienced this to a greater extent than others, but half of the dozen or so men interviewed seem to think this problem was significant in their daily lives. So, while this seemed to be a common problem in all men who were treated, it appeared worse in men who had had radical surgery for prostate gland removal. But, the brachytherapy and E-Beam PC patients interviewed voiced a similar lament: a high percentage of men (7 out of 12) had difficulty with urination because the penis seems to 'retreat' to the point that urination became an embarrassing event with soaked underware and pants.

There doesn't seem to be a particular treatment that makes this problem worse nor does it seem to effect a particular aged man, but it is worth noting that these after-effects of whatever treatment you choose for your PC will have some probability of occurring; to what extent it will effect YOU is impossible to predict but you need to know the 'shortening' of the penis is a by-product of whatever treatment you choose to get. And, it's a subject which is unlikely that your urologist or radiation oncologist will discuss, so be aware!

As noted elsewhere in this book, having a helpful and cooperating mate will be an important part of living with whatever after-effects of PC treatment may effect you. Overall, it appears that despite all the hype about nerve-sparing robotic radical surgery techniques, it is highly likely that men who have the prostate gland removed will have the most after-effects: sexual dysfunction for months and/or years following, incontinence for months or years following, and urination "issues" that may relate to the decrease "length" of the penis and the penis' tendency to 'retreat' making urination events difficult.

For all other treatments, varying degrees of after-effects are likely: frequent urination accompanied by burning sensations from mild to intense in the urethra and through the length of the penis will occur for months or years following treatment. The length of the penis will be reduced but sexual function is achievable within a week or two of treatment, with no loss of rigidity (although a stimulation aid may still be useful in the initial weeks after treatment). Again, a helpful mate/partner who understands what to do to help will greatly benefit the man who undergoes a non-surgical PC treatment regime. Just realize that it is likely that good sex and good urination with no incontinence, will be the most likely outcome for this PC treatment regime! Bon Appâtée...

So, now you have the tools necessary to make good treatment decisions. Your prostate health and your future happiness is in your hands now and I am confident the decisions you will make will ensure a long and healthy life. And, thank you for choosing Prostate Cancer 2.0 to help you with your decision-making process.

FINAL NOTES: Don't Take Newspaper Accounts As Gospel

Every time someone "famous" learns they have Prostate Cancer or divulges to the press that they will be treated for Prostate Cancer, the newspapers bring the disease into the public's view once more. Recent examples include former New York City mayor, Rudy Gulliani, Senator (and Presidential-wannabe) John Kerry, and (former) Secretary of State Colin Powell. Recently, billionaire Warren Buffet announced (April 2012) that he has 'stage II' PC (which is the first time I have heard PC described in 'stages' like other cancers...), and that he will delay treatment until mid-summer, since..." his doctor's indicated he's got time and he's not in immediate danger..." One assumes that means he's likely to get some type of radiation treatment (rather than a radical prostatectomy), but the point here is, famous people always get press and you should not be swayed by whatever the latest news-personality profile is on the treatment option you choose.

Always accompanying those press announcements, (except, so far, in Buffet's case), there is a brief discussion of the "treatment" that the individual chose and a review of statistics of the disease, but the information usually is almost always summarized in a manner that downplays the seriousness with which choice of treatment should be addressed. For instance, in both Kerry and Powell's cases, the press reported that..."*surgery would result in a complete cure and they would be back on the political treadmill in a matter of days with no noticeable after-effects...*"

In Powell's case, articles appeared in the same newspaper that described what a prostatectomy involves and quoted statistics that separated men by age into categories. The article noted that, seventy-five percent of those men over age 70 will have sexual dysfunction (no erection capability) while only one-third of those men under 50 who have their prostate gland removed will lose sexual capability! No word on the men between 50 and 70 years of age who choose radical prostatectomy, yet that's the largest age group diagnosed!

In addition, the press seems to extol the virtues of surgery for men who detect the disease in the early stages (i.e. before there is evidence it has spread outside the gland) on the basis that lymph nodes in the groin area can be removed at the same time, during the prostatectomy, and tested. It is presented very subtly but, for the uneducated and uninformed reader, the implication is (once again!) that getting the organ removed guarantees the cure!

By now, if you have been paying attention throughout this Edition 2.0, you have learned to read between the lines about any and all things medical. And, once again, it is clear that news from our media should reinforce the two messages that this book is hoping to make clear:

1.) Younger and younger men are being diagnosed with Prostate Cancer so beginning the PSA and DRE screening needs to occur at age 45, or earlier for men who have a family history;

2.) A positive diagnosis means it is time to start researching treatment options, including (and, MOST important!) obtaining second and third opinions from urologists, brachytherapists, and other medical professionals who specialize in treating prostate cancer;

3.) ***"IF YOU HAVE BEEN DIAGNOSED WITH CANCER (ANY CANCER…NOT ONLY PROSTATE CANCER), YOU ABSOLUTELY MUST SEEK MORE THAN ONE MEDICAL OPINION ABOUT YOUR TREATMENT OPTIONS! AND, YOU ABSOLUTELY MUST SEEK OPINIONS FROM DIFFERENT TREATMENT SPECIALISTS: SURGERY, RADIATION, CRYOGENICS, ROBOTICS SURGERY; ETC."***

This final message is the same one we started this Edition 2.0 with--- With all the materials and references that have been provided, you should now realize that a diagnosis is not a death sentence BUT, only you can make choices that will determine what quality of life you have while you live with prostate cancer---I wish you the best of luck; live a long and happy life!

Nicholas R. Hild, PhD., Emeritus Professor

SOME OTHER REFERENCES....

Khalsa, Dharma Singh, Meditation As Medicine, Pocket Books, New York, NY, 2001

__, April 19, 02; *Tomatoes cut prostate cancer risk,* Arizona Republic (AP Release

Advertising Supplement, May 2, '02; Cancer Research, et al.; Arizona Republic (SF Examiner)

__, May 9, 02, *Cancer link to vaccine discovered*; Arizona Republic

__, March 5, 2002; Blood test for breast cancer sought; Arizona Republic (AP Release)

__, AP; May 21, 2002, Arizona Republic; pg A5

Carper, Jean, (1997); Miracle Cures, Harper-Collins, NY, NY

NCCN, www.national comprehensive cancer.......; 2001

__, April, '02, Vol 3, #2, *Quercetin May Be A Natural Treatment for Prostate Cancer*; Healthkeepers Magazine

Mattern, H., May 5, '02, *The world as Herb sees it*; Arizona Republic

O'Hara, M.; (2001); Prostate Cancer Battle: It's Strictly Your Decision, 1st Books Online (at 1stbooks.com)

__. www.MayoClinic.com; 2001-2002

__, July, 2001; *Your Prostate Health* (Newsletter), Grado – Ragde Clinics, (distributed sporadically throughout the year to the medical community)

Goodman, Jack M., (1997), *"Prostate Cancer: Some Things Every Man Should Know* (Brochure), Available from VIVUS, Inc, 4469 W. Avalon, Phoenix, AZ 85031

Sheldon, S; Cedars Sinia Hospital (personal interview), April, 2001

The Healthy Cell News, Spring 2002, *"You Can Prevent and Even Stop Prostate Problems,"* ALV Publishers, Inc., PO Box 250, Young, AZ 85554

AARP Bulletin/January 2003; July/Aug 2003; (www.aarp.org/bulletin)

Clapp, Larry; Prostate Health in 90 Days, 9th printing-Feb. '99, Hay House, Inc., Carlsbad, CA.

Schachter, Michael, M.D., www.World Health OnLine (2001-2002)

Prostate: For Men and Women Who Care About Them, Today's Arizona Woman, June 2002

Bostwick, D., MacLennan, G., and Larson, T.; Prostate Cancer-What Every Man – And His Family - Should Know; 1996, (American Cancer Society); Random House, Inc.; NY, NY

US News & World Report, *Cancer: New Promise For Early Detection,* Vol 132, No. 22, June 24, 2002, pp 48-58

National Prostate Cancer Council (NPCC.com); June 2002

Hsing, Ann W., Journal of the National Cancer Institute, (Arizona Republic, October 15, 2002

Evans, Mark, *Gene Tied to Deadly Prostate Cancer*, October 9, 2002, AP Wire Story; http://apnews.excite.com/article/20021009/D7MI76EO0. html

(www.letstalkhealth.com); Newsletter (Vol 5, #3: Oct/Nov 2002); 1229 3rd Ave, Ste. C; Chula Vista, CA 91911

www.Yahoo! News – Viagra; Reuter News Limited, (Accessed) April 28, 2003

New England Journal of Medicine, I. Thompson, PI, June, 2003

Carper, J., *Eat Smart, High-Protein Hazards*; USA Weekend Magazine (usaweekend.com); Jul 4-6, 2003; pp 4.

Wentworth, R., (2002), Caught With My Pants Down, 1st Books Online at 1stbooks.com

__ JonssonCenter.com; (Aug03)"Update on Herbal and Alternative Medicine Research, (Internet Web Site for UCLA Cancer Research Center); Fall 2003

Cancer Epidemiology, *Biomarkers Previews.* 17: 80, 2008

Nutrition Action Healthletter, September 2008, Vol 35, Number 7, Center For Science in the Public Interest, M. Jacobson, PhD., Editor; Wash D.C.

Lawrence Livermore Labs; Cancer Research. 65: 11779, 2005

Wellness Letter, University of California, Berkeley, Vol. 24, Issue 12; September 2008

AUA Foundation, the Official Foundation of the American Urological Association, (ProstateCancerWatch.com), 2009

Cancer Letter, Clarke, J.D., Dashwood, R. H., and Ho, E. Multi-targeted prevention of cancer by sulforaphane; 269:291-304, 2008

Proceedings of National Academy of Science U.S.A., Frei, B. & Lawson,S., Vitamin C and cancer revisited, 105:11,037-11,038, 2008

Carcinogenesis, Nian, H, Delage, B., Pinto, J.T., and Dashwood, R. H., 29:1816-1824, 2008

Carcinogenesis, Nian, H., Bisson, W.H., Dashwood, W.M., Pinto, J.T., Dashwood, R.H., 30:1416-1423, 2009

Journal of Nutritional Biochemistry, Yan, M., Hardin, K, and Ho, E., zinc-induced apoptosis in BPH and prostate cancer cells, 2009

Research Newsletter of the Linus Pauling Institute, Fall/Winter 2009, www.lpi@oregonstate.edu (retrieved December 2009)

Made in the USA
Monee, IL
05 November 2026

67383321R00083